Praise for *Working With Grieving and Tr*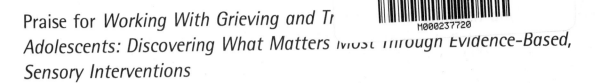 *Adolescents: Discovering What Matters Most Through Evidence-Based, Sensory Interventions*

"In the sea of rhetoric about trauma-informed care, *What Matters Most* delivers answers that will make a difference to young people right now. This book equips professionals working at all levels with young people impacted by trauma to do their work differently, incorporating one fundamental principle that stands above all else: this work is not about doing to children, but being with children, and empowering them in their own healing journey. From neuroscience to relational practice, this book is the most compelling and practical story about trauma treatment told to date."

—Kiaras Gharabaghi, PhD, Ryerson University, Toronto, Canada

"This book is a page-turner, a comment usually reserved for action novels. Rich with recent neuroscience findings, the impact of trauma on the brain, case studies, and specific interventions, *Working with Grieving and Traumatized Children and Adolescents* is a must-have resource for anyone who works with and cares about young people of any age. As a foster care survivor and now a college professor, I am grateful for Steele and Kuban's contribution."

—John Seita, EdD, School of Social Work, Michigan State University

"Building on years of developing and researching structured sensory interventions, the authors share poignant stories of resilience, integrate findings from neuroscience and empirical studies, and offer simple and effective interventions that build safe and secure relationships for grieving and traumatized children and teens."

—Anne L. Stewart, PhD, Professor of Graduate Psychology,
James Madison University, and president of the Virginia Association for Play Therapy

WORKING WITH GRIEVING AND TRAUMATIZED CHILDREN AND ADOLESCENTS

WORKING WITH GRIEVING AND TRAUMATIZED CHILDREN AND ADOLESCENTS

DISCOVERING WHAT MATTERS MOST THROUGH EVIDENCE-BASED, SENSORY INTERVENTIONS

WILLIAM STEELE
CAELAN KUBAN

WILEY

Cover Design: Wiley
Cover Image: © iStockphoto.com/Ron_Thomas

This book is printed on acid-free paper. ∞

Copyright © 2013 by John Wiley & Sons, Inc. All rights reserved.

Published by John Wiley & Sons, Inc., Hoboken, New Jersey.
Published simultaneously in Canada.

For general information on our other products and services, please contact our Customer Care Department within the United States at (800) 762-2974, outside the United States at (317) 572-3993 or fax (317) 572-4002.

Wiley publishes in a variety of print and electronic formats and by print-on-demand. Some material included with standard print versions of this book may not be included in e-books or in print-on-demand. If this book refers to media such as a CD or DVD that is not included in the version you purchased, you may download this material at http://booksupport.wiley.com. For more information about Wiley products, visit www.wiley.com.

Library of Congress Cataloging-in-Publication Data:

Steele, William.
    Working with grieving and traumatized children and adolescents : discovering what matters most through evidence-based, sensory interventions / William Steele, Caelan Kuban.
       1 online resource.
    Includes bibliographical references and index.
    Description based on print version record and CIP data provided by publisher; resource not viewed.
    ISBN 978-1-118-54317-7 (pbk)
    ISBN 978-1-118-64510-9 (ebk)
    ISBN 978-1-118-64507-9 (ebk)
      1. Grief in children.   2. Bereavement in children.   3. Loss (Psychology)   I. Kuban, Caelan.   II. Title.
BF723.G75
362.74—dc23

                                     2013004990

Printed in the United States of America
10 9 8 7 6 5 4 3 2 1

WILLIAM STEELE

To the resilient forces in my life:
my wife, son, and daughter, our grandchildren, and the thousands of professionals
I have met over the years, who continue to expect the best of themselves
in order to foster the strengths and resilience
of the grieving and traumatized children they are helping every day.

CAELAN KUBAN

To my daughters, Luscia and Maren,
who have allowed me to experience connection, joy, and love.
To my mother, Bridget, who gave me
not only her sunny disposition but also her unconditional support.
And to the many professionals whose time and expertise
have enhanced my understanding of what matters most
in our efforts to help grieving and traumatized children flourish.

Contents

Foreword

Reading *Working With Grieving and Traumatized Children and Adolescents* is like being blessed with having two wise, seasoned trauma therapists to consult whenever one is in need of support, encouragement, and inspiration. As Bill Steele, founder of the National Institute for Trauma and Loss in Children (TLC), and Caelan Kuban, current director of TLC, emphasize throughout this fine book, their clients have taught them much during their years of practice. Fortunately for the rest of us, the authors have decided to pay it forward by sharing these lessons of hope and resilience with readers.

What I love about this book is that the authors have created a reading experience for us that actually parallels the process of the therapeutic relationship they create with their clients. One indispensable quality of effective therapy is authenticity, and as I read the book, I encountered real people—clients, parents, teachers, and therapists—in every chapter. I was not reading the typical, traditional case studies that characterize so many books on therapy. Those case studies often strike me as formulaic, contrived, analytical, and superficial. They leave me perhaps edified, but rarely moved. Instead, in *Working With Grieving and Traumatized Children and Adolescents*, I experienced narratives that were told with all the vivid characterizations and dramatic power of short stories. These rich and nuanced accounts rang true in their depth, authenticity, and complexity. They did much more than demonstrate principles; they touched me, stirred my emotions, invited me to care deeply, and ultimately inspired me. By engaging us with such powerful illustrations and narratives, the authors do much more than help us understand important concepts and principles. At a deep and implicit level, we truly get it.

I also love that the book dedicates an entire chapter to the topic of curiosity and celebrates taking the stance of not knowing. As a trainer of therapists, I have discovered that students find it particularly challenging to accept not knowing as an essential condition for successful therapy. After all, aren't they attending graduate school, studying diligently, and earning their degrees in order to become *experts*? Setting aside that professional mask and stepping down from that expert pedestal to encounter our clients, to learn from them, and to bear witness to their journey of healing are daunting tasks. However, once students follow the example of Steele and Kuban by taking these risks, they can engage in their own transformative experiences of *being* truly therapeutic—not merely *doing* therapy.

Another parallel between the book and the process of therapy is that each chapter of *Working With Grieving and Traumatized Children and Adolescents* begins and ends in a safe place—just like a successful session. Steele and Kuban also practice what they preach by following the show-and-tell method of their therapy. They first share with us the powerful drawings by clients that give expression to the raw, searing experience of their traumas. The authors then elaborate on these pictures by using words to give voice to their therapeutic narratives.

One particularly disturbing case study reminded me of the classic Harry Harlow studies (1958) on infant rhesus macaque monkeys who were separated from their mothers. Virtually every introductory psychology textbook contains stunning pictures of these poor, traumatized creatures, clinging desperately to their cloth surrogate mothers. What is little known, however, is that a later study, reported by Cozolino (2010), demonstrated that these monkeys were not condemned to a life of profound dysfunction and alienation. In fact, Harlow and Suomi (1971) developed a successful therapy, involving 12 sessions, for these deeply troubled monkeys! The therapists were other monkeys who had been raised with healthy attachments. Although these monkeys were smaller and welcoming, the isolated "clients" reacted with anxiety whenever the "therapists" at first tried to engage with them. However, the gentle touches and persistent overtures of the "therapists" won out as the "clients" began to feel safe and began to interact with them. At the conclusion of the therapy, the initially isolated monkeys successfully joined the colony. I'm willing to bet that most practitioners believed that these monkeys were hopeless cases. Steele and Kuban have dedicated their professional lives to working with similarly supposed hopeless cases and to sharing their invitational, gentle, and nonthreatening manner of drawing out the strengths and nurturing the resilience of their clients.

An unexpected bonus of this book is that readers also gain a greater understanding of neuroscience, including mirror neurons, brain functioning, neural plasticity, and neural pathways. Steele and Kuban artfully introduce neuroscience principles and research findings in the context of their dramatic narratives of trauma and triumph. As a result, instead of inflicting on us a dry treatise on brain functioning, the authors engage us in a mystery in which neuroscience is providing clues into what makes our clients—and us!—tick.

Based on the work of Cozolino (2010) and other neuroscientists, Steele and Kuban highlight how empathic attunement, which is the foundation for a safe and secure relationship, promotes neural plasticity. Such a therapeutic alliance, which activates the processes of attachment, is the optimal chemical environment for creating new neural pathways. They practice a therapy that is based on synchrony and attunement. One of the common slogans of neuroscientists is, "Neurons that fire together, wire together." In other words, therapy invites the creative expression of previously dissociated, denied, or inhibited thoughts and feelings. This process of working through experiences builds new neural pathways.

Building on the fundamental insight that therapy is a shared here-and-now experience, Steele and Kuban have developed wonderfully creative techniques to help clients express their experiences in modalities other than verbal communication. By immersing their clients in the creative moment and expanding their awareness, Steele and Kuban have enabled traumatized, grieving children and youth to create narratives of resilience and transcendence.

I would also like to mention that the timing of this publication is fortuitous. As the publication of *DSM-5* approaches, numerous articles have been written on proposed changes to the PTSD diagnosis. Ever since PTSD was entered into the official psychiatric nosology in 1980, "no other psychiatric diagnosis, with the exception of Dissociative Identity Disorder (a related disorder), has generated so much controversy in the field as to the boundaries of the disorder, diagnostic criteria, central assumptions, clinical utility, and prevalence in various populations" (Spitzer, First, & Wakefield, 2007). In *Working With Grieving and Traumatized Children and Adolescents*, Steele and Kuban provide a convincing argument for adding a new diagnosis, Developmental Trauma Disorder (DTD), in the *DSM-5* (van der Kolk & Pynoos, 2009). The proposal of this diagnosis was based on the findings from developmental psychopathology, the clinical presentations of children and youth exposed to chronic interpersonal violence, and emerging evidence from the field of neurobiology regarding the impact of trauma on brain development. They note that the *DSM* PTSD criteria were not developmentally sensitive and did not capture clinically relevant symptoms for children living in chronically unsafe conditions. However, the proposed PTSD criteria for *DSM-5* would result in inaccurate diagnoses for children who undergo multiple and complex traumas, especially those exposed to harmful caregiving (van der Kolk & Pynoos, 2009). The proposal for DTD was not accepted for inclusion in *DSM-5*, but thanks to Steele and Kuban, the discussion of the merits of an alternative classification system for children experiencing complex trauma is continuing.

Working With Grieving and Traumatized Children and Adolescents includes many "magical moments" of therapy that practitioners have described to the authors with heartfelt eloquence. Interestingly, in addition to studying the work of therapists, researchers are now beginning to investigate how stage magicians exploit neuroscience to create their illusions. In other words, magicians are just as much practitioners of sleight of mind (Macknik & Martinez-Conde, 2010) as they are of sleight of hand. Although magicians take advantage of neurological processes to trick audiences, therapists use the same processes to enhance neuroplasticity. Consequently, a magic performance can leave a spectator mystified, but therapy can leave a traumatized client transformed.

Speaking of magic, the authors pull off a great trick themselves with this book. While giving detailed instructions and excellent examples of how to help clients reframe their experiences of trauma, Steele and Kuban skillfully guide us readers into reframing our own roles as trauma therapists. By the time we finish their book, we have come to cherish the power of curiosity as a powerful therapeutic tool, to respect the transformative potential of bearing witness rather than dispensing expertise, and to focus on what's strong rather than what's wrong with a client. Now, that's a magic moment!

Lennis G. Echterling
James Madison University

References

Cozolino, L. (2010). *The neuroscience of psychotherapy: Healing the social brain* (2nd ed.). New York, NY: W. W. Norton.

Harlow, H. F. (1958). The nature of love. *American Psychologist, 13,* 673–685.

Harlow, H. F., & Suomi, S. J. (1971). Social recovery by isolation-reared monkeys. *Proceedings of the National Academy of Sciences, USA, 68,* 1534–1538.

Macknik, S. L., & Martinez-Conde, S. (2010). *Sleights of mind: What the neuroscience of magic reveals about our everyday deceptions.* New York, NY: Picador.

Spitzer, R. L., First, M. B., & Wakefield, J. C. (2007). Saving PTSD from itself in DSM-5. *Journal of Anxiety Disorders, 21,* 233–241. doi: 10.1016/j.janxdis.2006.09.006

van der Kolk, B. A., & Pynoos, R. (2009). Proposal to include a developmental trauma disorder diagnosis for children and adolescents in *DSM-5.* Retrieved from www.traumacenter.org/announcements/DTD_papers_Oct_09.pdf

Preface

The mandate coming from both grieving and traumatized children today is to spend time in their world—a sensory world without language—to see what they actually see when they look at themselves, others, and the world as a result of what they have experienced. From their perspective, if we cannot see what they see, feel what they feel, and think what they think, how can we possibly know what matters most in their efforts to remain resilient and flourish despite the troubling and traumatic situations they experience?

The following experiences, and many others, represent the kind of grief- and trauma-inducing situations; varied levels of severity, complexity, and diverse environments; and developmental ranges of children and adolescents that have taught us so much over the past 22 years:

➤ The parents of a 4-year-old daughter and 6-year-old son divorce. The son is managing fairly well, whereas the daughter struggles with nightmares and has become very defiant.

➤ An only daughter, 8 years old, witnesses her mother dying from cancer at home. One year later she has isolated herself, is quite sad, and is still very fearful and traumatized by all the sensory memories of her mother's physical and emotional deterioration.

➤ At age 2, Alex witnesses his father kill his mother. Now age 7, the only way he can fall asleep is to sleep on the floor.

➤ Taken from his mother at an early age, James is moved in and out of 15 different foster care homes.

➤ Three siblings, ages 5, 11, and 15, are traumatized by the brutal rape and murder of their stepsister. One year later, all of them are involved in challenging and troublesome behavior.

➤ Abused, neglected, and raped multiple times, 15-year-old Ruby has become unmanageable.

> A mother and her 4-year-old son drive up to their garage. As the mother opens the garage door, both are struck with terror as they see the body of the boy's father hanging dead.

> Two teenagers are killed in an auto accident, while four friends following in the car behind them witness it all.

> While bending over to catch the baseball his 7-year-old grandson hit, the boy's grandfather dies suddenly of a heart attack.

> Twenty-four high school students witness the shooting and murder of their beloved coach. Months later, they and their parents are struggling at home and at school with intense fears, worries, and emotions that alter their relationships and ability to perform.

> A high school student stabs his teacher to death in the classroom. Parents, staff, and students are overwhelmed.

> The many victims of the Gulf War, the bombing of the Federal Building in Oklaholma City, 9/11, and Hurricanes Katrina and Rita continue to deal with the aftermath of these events.

By presenting these survivors with opportunities to bring us into their troubling and traumatic worlds, to see what they saw as they looked at themselves and the world around them, to discover what was driving their challenging behaviors, we learned to abandon traditional intervention processes for structured, sensory-based experiences that evidence-based outcomes and practice history now demonstrate are effective in reducing posttraumatic stress and related mental health symptoms and behaviors.

Advances in neuroscience clearly support rethinking our understanding of grief and trauma and the interventions we practice. The five stages of grief, for example, developed in the late 1960s by Dr. Elisabeth Kubler-Ross, have been used for years to guide the treatment of grief. Today these stages are axiomatic, no longer reflecting the reality of how grief is experienced and processed. Furthermore, neuroscience has clearly documented that trauma is not primarily a cognitive experience but a series of subjective experiences that do not respond well to our use of reason, logic, or talk-based interventions. These advances alter the way we must relate with grieving and traumatized children today.

Becoming a witness to these subjective experiences and helping survivors transform their internal grieving and trauma-specific implicit memories and sensations into concrete, tangible forms in ways that lead to the restoration of their sense of safety, empowerment, and resilience are the strategies we detail in *Working With Grieving and Traumatized Children and Adolescents*.

A Timely Practical Resource

The detailed, evidence-based intervention strategies we present make this a timely, practical resource for addressing the realities of today's grieving and traumatized children, adolescents, and adults in schools, agencies, and clinical and community settings. The intervention model presented, *SITCAP®* (*Structured Sensory Interventions for Traumatized Children, Adolescents and Parents*), was developed in 1990 by the National Institute for Trauma and Loss in Children (TLC), a nonprofit program of the Starr Global Learning Network, which has been helping children and adolescents flourish for more than 100 years.

Benefiting Survivors and Practitioners in Diverse Settings

Several aspects make *Working With Grieving and Traumatized Children and Adolescents* unique:

➤ It is based on the TLC's 23 years of working with grieving and traumatized children, families, and professionals in school, agency, and community-based programs across the country.

➤ The *SITCAP* intervention model has met the criteria for best practices (practice-based evidence) as supported by consistent outcomes over years of practice by 6,000 TLC Certified Trauma and Loss Specialists and by published, formal evidence-based research conducted in school and agency settings.

➤ The interventions have been demonstrated to address violent situations, such as murder, physical and sexual abuse, and domestic violence, as well as nonviolent grief- and trauma-inducing situations, such as divorce, critical injuries, car fatalities, terminal illness, and environmental disasters.

➤ Each chapter provides activities for use when helping children with specific aspects of their subjective experiences, such as terror, worry, guilt, and powerlessness. In addition, each chapter includes a brief *Point of Interest* insert that addresses specific topic areas such as Attention Deficit Hyperactive Disorder and PTSD and *Magical Moments*, the key turning points for children as told by practitioners using *SITCAP* with children and adolescents.

➤ Given that services for grieving and traumatized children and families are severely shrinking, while waiting lists are extended for months, *Working With Grieving and Traumatized Children and Adolescents* provides practitioners the opportunity to safely apply very structured, sensory- and evidence-based, short-term interventions that have demonstrated long-term gains.

➤ *Working With Grieving and Traumatized Children and Adolescents* approaches healing within the parameters of the more recent findings regarding the resilience of those who are exposed to significant losses or trauma, as well as what children, when given the opportunity, tell us matters the most to their healing, recovery, and resilience.

➤ The use of *SITCAP* is supported by ongoing training conducted by TLC, its manualized programs inclusive of developmentally appropriate workbooks with activity worksheets that can be copied, additional resource materials that address specific issues involving grief and trauma, numerous continuing education approved online courses, and easy access to TLC, its staff, and Certified Trauma Practitioners.

For the Reader

Through the use of vivid characterizations, dramatic short stories, sequential and structured processes, and the integration of training activities used in actual training in the use of the *SITCAP* model, readers will learn:

➤ Why children's experiences, rather than symptoms and behaviors, matter significantly in determining what will be most helpful to their healing

➤ Ways to be *curious* rather than *analytical* to allow children to safely bring us into their secret, often terrifying worlds, while revealing the private logic driving their grief- and trauma-related behaviors

➤ What is meant by *sensory-based interventions* and how they can help children reveal what they are thinking, feeling, and now seeing when they look at themselves and the world around them, when they have neither the words nor the language to describe their thoughts, feelings, view of self, and others (activities will be presented)

➤ How to apply intervention to the 10 primary experiences of trauma and grief

➤ The critical timelines used to determine the most appropriate interventions with grieving and traumatized children within a school setting

➤ How to determine the gains made by children when a formal assessment is not available

➤ How we help children create narratives of resilience and strengths, which help them begin to flourish

➤ What allows some children to do better than others who are exposed to the same situation and the kinds of interactions that help them maintain resilience even in the face of future grief- and trauma-inducing situations

We hope that the *Magical Moments* shared by practitioners in this text and the structured intervention processes we present on our journey into the world of the children's stories we tell reveal that what matters most in our efforts to help is our ability to provide them with the opportunity to make us a witness to how they are experiencing themselves and their world, while teaching us what matters most to their ongoing efforts to flourish despite the significant losses and trauma they have experienced so young in life.

William Steele
Caelan Kuban

Acknowledgments

We wish to acknowledge Starr Commonwealth and the Starr Global Learning Network staff for their ongoing efforts to help us create practices that help children flourish and for affording us the time needed to prepare this work. Special thanks goes to Deva Ludwig, for all of the technical support and creative encouragement she provided, and to Sarah Slamer, whose assistance with preparing case material was invaluable. We thank Deanne Ginns-Gruenberg, owner of the Self Esteem Bookstore, for allowing us hours and hours to review and learn from the many books authored by others in the field. Naomi Chedd, Licensed Mental Health Counselor and Educational Consultant, in Brookline, Massachusettts, provided a most helpful review and critique of the manuscript. The expertise, support, and recommendations of Rachael Livsey, Senior Editor at John Wiley & Sons provided to us throughout the development and completion of this work were invaluable.

Over the past 20 years, we have had the wonderful opportunity to learn a great deal from thousands of traumatized children and their families. In many ways, they are the authors of this book. We cannot thank them enough for their inspiration, resilience, and guidance in defining what matters most in our efforts to help children heal from grief and trauma. Hundreds of dedicated professionals also volunteered their time to participate in field testing and rigorous research of our evidence-based sensory intervention programs. Their feedback ensured that the intervention processes and activities accomplished what they were intended to accomplish: significant reduction of PTSD and other mental health–related reactions while strengthening the resilience of grieving and traumatized children. We thank them for all of the valuable lessons they have taught us over the years. We also wish to acknowledge the hundreds of school districts, child care agencies, and mental health and community-based programs that have collaborated with us to bring best practices to the grieving and traumatized children, adolescents, and families they serve every day. Their efforts are making a difference.

CHAPTER One

How Structured, Sensory Interventions Help Grieving and Traumatized Children

This first chapter begins with a brief history of what we learned at the National Institute for Trauma and Loss in Children (TLC) while working with grieving and traumatized children who had been exposed to a variety of violent and nonviolent experiences. Established in 1990, TLC is a program of the Starr Global Learning Network of Starr Commonwealth, which has been helping children and adolescents flourish for the past 100 years. The children taught us what mattered most in their efforts to overcome their painful and overwhelming experiences, which lead to the development of the evidence-based *Structured Sensory Interventions for Children, Adolescents and Parents* (*SITCAP*) programs presented in detail in this text. The *SITCAP* model meets the criteria validating it as a practice-based and an evidence-based intervention model. This criteria and how it is supported by *SITCAP* is reviewed, as funding sources are more frequently requesting that today's interventions meet these requirements.

In addition, a distinction is made between nonviolent and violent situations to illustrate that the subjective experiences of children, not the nature of the situation, determine whether the experiences are grief or trauma inducing. This is followed by a very simple yet profound mandate by children and a brief discussion regarding its implications for treatment. This introduction becomes essential to understanding the *Core Principle* and *Key Concepts* of *SITCAP* presented in subsequent chapters. These concepts describe how children's subjective experiences are revealed and utilized to help diminish the painful, overwhelming, and terrifying reactions they can experience. Similar to Lenore Terr's (2008) descriptions of magical moments in psychotherapy, we also introduce *Magical Moments*, those turning points in children's lives that practitioners using *SITCAP* shared with us over the years. *Magical Moments* are featured in each chapter, in addition to *Points of Interest*, which briefly discuss a variety of subjects pertinent to helping grieving and traumatized children and adolescents. The chapter concludes with a review of two cases and their evidence-based outcomes, supporting the overall benefits experienced by those who have participated in *SITCAP* over the years.

Was It Grief or Trauma: What Matters Most?

Examining our experiences in the 1970s and 1980s with children, teens, and families who sought help while in crisis—or created a crisis to draw attention to their need for help—revealed what mattered most in our efforts to help. Grief was a common response to their crisis experiences resulting from the losses precipitating their crises—loss involving a loved one to sudden or accidental death, suicide, homicide, domestic violence, sexual and physical abuse, or terminal illness, or loss due to divorce, betrayal of trust in relationships, abandonment, homelessness, or exposure to catastrophic events. In the early 1980s, suicide became an epidemic claiming the lives of youth. At the core of the suicide experience is the loss of value for oneself, the loss of connectedness to any significant person, and the loss created for the family members and friends who are left behind. In the later 1980s, suicide rates remained high; however, violence claimed this unfortunate title of epidemic, reflecting the disturbing ways our children were now experiencing their worlds.

With these losses, we were observing reactions not only associated with grief but also with the posttraumatic stress disorder (PTSD) described in the *Diagnostic and Statistical Manual of Mental Disorders* (*DSM-III-R*) (APA, 1980). Unfortunately, these criteria, as defined by the *DSM-III-R*, were specific to adults. The challenge we faced was helping others acknowledge that children could, in fact, experience the reactions attributed to adults at the time. This would not occur until the mid-1990s. Practitioners in the 1980s, for example, observed adult PTSD criteria in adolescent survivors of suicide as well as those who discovered the bodies of those who took their own lives. However, it wasn't until 1993 and subsequent years that the literature began to acknowledge that discovering the body of a loved one, friend, or peer who had taken their life was traumatic (Brent et al., 1993). The term *trauma* was not formally assigned to children by the American Psychological Association until 1994, when they were included in the adult-designed PTSD diagnostic category in the *DSM-IV* (APA, 1994). This inclusion was certainly encouraged by the research that emerged in the 1980s regarding the association of PTSD with suicide and violence among children and adolescents (Pynoos & Eth, 1986; Pynoos et al., 1987).

Despite the various situations that brought children and families to our attention, so many victims showed us that grief and trauma were not necessarily separate entities; they often coexisted. Symptoms could be attributed to both grief and trauma, as we understood them at that time, but also to other disorders, making it difficult to assign treatment based on symptoms alone. What we discovered really mattered the most to those who were grieving and traumatized was *not their symptoms, but how they experienced themselves, others, and life following exposure to traumatic events in their lives.* TLC was founded in 1990 to develop an intervention process that would be helpful to both grieving and traumatized children and that could be initiated in clinical and community settings and also in schools, where children are the most accessible.

It Is Not the Situation

An Internet search for *trauma-informed care* yields more than 7 million references. It is safe to say that a great deal of information exists about the prevalence of trauma experienced by children and what constitutes trauma-informed care. The majority of articles regarding trauma consistently cite violence as the primary cause of trauma. There is no doubt that violence does induce severe trauma in children. Most would agree that at least 50% of the children in child welfare and 60% to 70% of youth in the juvenile justice system experience trauma (Hodas, 2006; Kerig & Becker, 2010). However, research began to emerge as early as the 1990s indicating that trauma can also be induced by disasters such as fires (McFarlane, Policansky, & Irwin, 1987), hurricanes (Lonigan, Shannon, Finch, Daugherty, & Taylor, 1991), boating accidents (Yule, 1992), burns, and medical procedures such as bone marrow transplants (Stubner, Nader, Yasuda, Pynoos, & Cohen, 1991). Three million people yearly are involved in car accidents; up to 45% of those injured suffer PTSD (Goodin & Abernathy, 2011). In fact, divorce can also induce trauma when the conditions of that experience leave children vulnerable (Divorce and PTSD, 2012).

We have two reasons for making this distinction between violent and nonviolent situations, which are not the result of direct intent to do harm. First, in comparison to the volumes written about the relationship between violence and trauma, we rarely read about the daily nonviolent trauma-inducing situations in children, such as homelessness. Often, trauma is not screened for in children who are exposed to situations such as a depressed parent, house fires, car fatalities, critical injuries, terminal illnesses, divorce, or victims of bullying and cyber bullying. Second, we must conclude that if both violent and nonviolent situations can induce trauma, then perhaps it is not the situation that induces trauma but how that situation is being experienced that leaves children and youth vulnerable to trauma. If this is true, then it follows that we must first know how children are experiencing what they are exposed to if we want to determine what might be the most helpful and appropriate trauma-informed response.

Children's Mandate

If you don't think what I think, feel what I feel, experience what I experience, and see what I see when I look at myself, others, and the world around me, how can you possibly know what is best for me?

This is a simple yet profoundly wise mandate. When we can appreciate how traumatized children are experiencing themselves, others, and their lives as a result of their experiences, we can assign timely, useful, and appropriate interventions. Resilience research, for example, clearly documents that not everyone exposed to what we might consider to be a trauma-inducing incident is necessarily traumatized by that incident

(Bonanno et al., 2002). Assigning an appropriate intervention dictates that we first determine how children are experiencing what they are exposed to if we are to provide an intervention that is not itself traumatizing. In fact, the primary dictate of trauma-informed care is to avoid re-traumatizing, "to do no harm" (Hodas, 2006), by not making assumptions that children must be traumatized by what they have been exposed to or, if traumatized, that all children need the same intervention (Steele & Raider, 2001).

In essence, a situation such as divorce may not be violent or traumatizing for many children. However, even in a nonviolent divorce—one void of physical abuse and threats of bodily harm—if the child's experience of that divorce involves terror, worry, guilt, feeling powerless, and other subjective experiences associated with trauma, then that divorce may become traumatic. This is why interventions must match how children are experiencing their life events.

Implications for Treatment

The child-driven mandate presented earlier dictates that to be helpful we need to relate to grieving and traumatized children at a sensory level rather than primarily at a cognitive level. What does this mean? Today neuroscience has confirmed that trauma is experienced in the midbrain, the limbic region, sometimes referred to as the "feeling" brain or the "survival" brain, where there is no reason, logic, or language. Reason, logic, and the use of language, to make sense of what has happened, are upper brain cognitive functions that become difficult to access in trauma (Brendtro, Mitchell, & McCall, 2009; Levine & Kline, 2008; Perry, 2009; Schore, 2001; van der Kolk, McFarlane, & Weisaeth, 1996). Neuroscience also shows that "learning anything requires building new neural networks [by] being actively involved in what is being learned" (Fischer, 2012).

For these reasons, we must direct our efforts at helping children with how they are experiencing their worlds, with what they now see when they look at themselves and others as a result of their exposure to trauma. We must engage them in nonverbal, sensory-based experiences that allow them to rework their traumatic memories and their trauma-related sensations, images, and feelings in ways that also allow them to see themselves and their experience as survivors and thrivers, not victims. We must help them to see and experience others as helpful and supportive rather than threatening and unsafe, and to see and experience life as promising rather than continually painful. This goal is difficult to accomplish using cognitive-based interventions alone. If, for example, I experienced something terrifying months earlier and I am now physically safe, but elements in my environment are reminding me of that terrifying experience (my midbrain is being activated by the associated memories), then all of the verbal reassurance in the world will not calm me. I must do something that brings about a sense of safety and calms (deactivates) my midbrain responses to those past memories. Numerous examples and sensory-based activities that restore this sense of safety are presented throughout the book.

A Magical Moment

My magical moment in using *SITCAP* is about a 7-year-old boy. He had lovely eyes with an eagerness and innocence that shone through. Much of his little life had been filled with turbulence and trauma. He had witnessed violence in his home and had experienced neglect and emotional abuse. In our work together, we had been using many interventions from *SITCAP* programs. In one session, Shawn (not his real name) was telling me how he would hear his mom and dad fight a lot. I asked if he could show me how that felt in his body when he thought about it now. He drew a picture of a person with a breaking heart and said he felt sad, scared, and worried. We talked about the meaning of each feeling for him and how he experienced it in his body. Then, spontaneously, he drew an image of a worry thermometer. He exclaimed that this thermometer goes from 0 to 100, and that his worries were so big that it was more than 100 degrees, and that the thermometer broke. "That's how much I worry!" he said.

Shawn then asked me to make a string of paper dolls. He took the paper dolls, and he drew happy faces on all seven of them and asked me to draw hearts on their bodies. He called these dolls the "worry breakers." He paid special attention to the doll on the far right, calling it "a soldier." He said that this soldier is the leader, and the rest of the dolls follow to help fight and break worries. As he spoke about the power of these dolls, his eyes widened and his back straightened. I could feel his own power growing as he spoke with confidence about how he might use these dolls in his life when he starts to feel worried. We then noticed the paper that was left over from cutting out the paper dolls looked like a crown. Shawn invited me to assist with drawing hearts and stars on the crown. We then stapled the ends together and, putting it on his head, he reported, "This crown helps with sad feelings!"

We talked about how he and his mom could use his powerful new resources. We walked around the room practicing how it felt to wear the crown and how that felt different in his body and could help with sad and scared feelings. Toward the end of our session, I looked at his picture of the thermometer again and asked if he could show me how he felt now. Shawn took another piece of paper and began drawing purposefully. As he put down his marker, he looked right at me, smiling with his bright green eyes and said, "This is an angel with wings. The angel is very special because it shoots love arrows to all people who need it." There was a calm presence about him.

As a therapist, *SITCAP* helps us create a safe holding space, guided by clear clinical interventions. Knowing our own therapeutic map allows us to step aside and let the magic begin to take shape. This little fellow knew what he needed to do. He was following his own magic inside—the kind of magic that allows a beautiful unfolding of a child's healing path as he journeys toward wholeness of spirit, body, and mind.

Carmen Richardson, MSW, RSW, RCAT, REAT
Prairie Institute of Expressive Arts Therapy, Calgary, Alberta, CANADA T3C 0P9

Subjective Experiences Matter

It is well argued and supported by abundant research that traumatized children today are going undiagnosed and misdiagnosed. Trauma symptoms are often mistaken for depression, attention deficit problems, oppositional defiant disorder (ODD), conduct disorder, reactive attachment, and other disorders (van der Kolk et al., 2009). This is partly because of our traditional focus on using symptoms and deficits as criteria for diagnosis, as well as the current, very narrow PTSD diagnosis found in the *DSM-IV-TR* (APA, 2000).

In 2005 and again in 2010, Robert Pynoos, Bessel van der Kolk, and their colleagues proposed a more relevant trauma category that reflects how traumatized children are presenting today and the abundant documentation neuroscience has provided regarding trauma's impact on the brain, the body, behavior, learning, and emotions. Although not included in the *DSM-5*, the proposed Developmental Trauma Disorder (DTD) presents a much more comprehensive, representative, and descriptive view of how traumatized children experience themselves, others, and the world around them as a result of their exposure to traumatic experiences (van der Kolk et al., 2009). It also puts those experiences within a developmental perspective, which is infrequently discussed in the literature. How a divorce is experienced at age 6, for example, is completely different than how it is experienced at age 16. Interventions must be different because of the developmental differences and experiences existing between these two age groups. This is also the case, for example, when a child is chronologically age 10 but developmentally more representative of a 6-year-old. At the time of this writing, the changes being made to the PTSD category in the *DSM-5* include (1) a preschool subtype for children ages 6 and under— Posttraumatic Stress Disorder in Preschool Children, (2) a dissociative subtype, and (3) a six-month requirement for children for the bereavement-related subtype (APA, 2012).

Although the proposed DTD category remains under consideration, its focus on the subjective experiences of trauma is critical to appreciating what matters most in our efforts to best understand and respond to traumatized children. In listing the prescribed criteria for exposure, the proposed DTD lists the following subjective experiences of traumatized children: rage, betrayal, fear, resignation, defeat, and shame. In other words, the experiences matter. TLC has always approached trauma as an experience rather than a diagnostic category. The evidence-based *SITCAP* programs of TLC address what we found in 1990 and continue to find today to be the common experiences associated with trauma: fear, terror, worry, hurt, anger, revenge, guilt/shame, feeling unsafe, powerless, and engaged in victim thinking versus survivor/thriver thinking (Steele & Raider, 2001). This listing is more detailed than those found in the proposed DTD, but it is certainly inclusive of those criteria. *SITCAP* interventions are therefore directed at these primary experiences and themes within a developmentally appropriate context. The following discussion of the Core Principle and Key Concepts is based on these early experiences with children, field testing, and evidence-based research that supports their value in the healing outcomes grieving and traumatized children have achieved.

Because trauma always involves significant losses, grief is part of the trauma experience (Levine & Kline, 2007). In subsequent chapters, we use the terms *trauma* and *traumatized children* with the understanding that we are also addressing the grief reactions inherent in the trauma response.

SITCAP's Core Principle

The core principle of the *SITCAP* model is that by providing children with the opportunity to safely revisit and rework the primary subjective experiences of trauma, within the sensory, not cognitive context in which they are experienced, stored, and remembered, PTSD symptoms and grief- and trauma-related mental health reactions can be significantly reduced, the gains sustained, and resilience developed and/or strengthened in ways that support growth.

We stated earlier that neuroscience has confirmed that trauma is experienced in the midbrain, where reason and logic—the ability to make sense of what has happened and act accordingly—simply are not accessible in trauma. Another way to explain how trauma is not primarily a cognitive experience is to examine memory processes, specifically the differences between *explicit* and *implicit* memory processes. Explicit memory, sometimes referred to as *declarative memory*, refers to primary cognitive processes in the neocortex region or the upper brain, also referred to as the left hemisphere. In explicit memory we have access to language; we have words to describe what we are thinking and feeling. Explicit memory allows us to process information, to reason, and to make sense of our experiences.

Such cognitive processes actually help us cope; however, trauma is experienced in implicit memory, sometimes referred to as the midbrain or right hemisphere, where there is no reason or language. There simply are no words to accurately describe or communicate what is being experienced. Positron emission tomography (PET) scans have found that trauma also creates changes in Broca's area of the brain, which leads to difficulties in identifying and verbalizing our experiences (Fosha, 2000; Van Dalen, 2001), a process that is normally accessible via explicit memory processes. In implicit memory, the traumatic memories are stored through our senses—what we see, hear, smell, touch, and taste (Rothschild, 2000).

If, therefore, there is no language to help children communicate what their experience is like, what matters most is that we present them with opportunities to communicate what it is like without words. The *SITCAP* process directs itself at actively involving children in new experiences in order for them to build new neural networks related to what they are learning about themselves and trauma as a result of the sensory-based activities they engage in when participating in *SITCAP*. The intervention process involves multiple sensory-based activities, which bring these sensory memories to life in a safe, contained context so they can be regulated, reordered, and reframed in ways that support a resilient response to future stressful, overwhelming, and terrifying experiences.

Point of Interest

SMAD!

While attending a recent conference, the presenter told a story about talking to a 4-year-old boy about labeling feelings. "Sometimes when we are sad, we cry and feel hurt, but at the same time we might be mad about something, too," is the statement that was told to the child. The 4-year-old responded, "Yeah, it's like being smad!"

Science supports this feeling, as described by the 4-year-old. In fact, Green, Whitney, and Potegal (2011) published a paper that details the patterned vocalizations that toddlers make during a tantrum. Sad sounds tend to occur throughout the entire tantrum, and on top of those sounds are typically sharp peaks of anger.

Learning the science behind a tantrum and understanding the pattern can help parents and professionals better respond to children. The stress that children experience when they have a tantrum shuts off the part of their brain that allows them to process, reason, and problem-solve. So, will asking children questions during tantrums help? Most likely the answer is no. It will make things worse, and the tantrum will ultimately last longer. Instead, stay with children through the peaks of anger, but don't try to reason with them. This means waiting through the screaming, yelling, kicking, pulling, and pushing without talking. The most important thing is to make sure they are safe. Once this peak is past, children will be left with sadness and will reach out for comfort. When this happens, comfort them with a hug, holding or sitting close beside them. Wait through the mad until you reach the sad!

Key Concepts

Subsequent chapters discuss in detail the ways neuroscience, resilience research and strength-based practices, and the key processes of trauma-informed care support these *SITCAP* intervention concepts.

Concept One: Safely Revisiting Subjective Experiences

Concept one is helping children safely revisit their traumatic experience(s) and/or work on those subjective experiences created by past exposures by focusing not on the trauma experience itself but on how they are experiencing themselves, others, and the varied environments they are attempting to navigate daily, but doing so with the primal survival behaviors associated with trauma.

The following key processes reported in *Trauma-Informed Practices for Children and Adolescents* (Steele & Malchiodi, 2012, p. 96) are incorporated into *SITCAP* to support it as a safe intervention for children as well as the practitioner. They include the following:

- Introduce choice and control
- Use a structured approach
- Be a witness rather than an analyst
- Be curious and use open-ended questions
- Teach children to be mindful of the sensations associated with interventions
- Instruct children to stop anytime interventions become too activating
- Instruct children to stop us when what we are asking is too activating
- Follow the pace children set and practice titration
- Begin the session in a safe place and end in a safe place
- Help children recognize the pleasant and unpleasant sensations in their bodies, always resourcing those pleasant sensations when children are experiencing unpleasant, activating sensations
- Incorporate appropriate strategies according to principles of neurodevelopment
- Repeat interventions used to regulate or deactivate children's trauma-related reactions frequently in order to help them discover they have the ability to regulate those reactions
- Identify and involve at least one adult with whom children are familiar to reinforce what is learned
- Keep in mind that children always remain the best experts about what is helping and what is hurting

The *SITCAP* programs also address what children have consistently indicated as their common subjective experiences associated with trauma: fear, terror, worry, hurt, anger, revenge, guilt/shame, feeling unsafe, powerless, and engaged in victim thinking versus survivor/thriver thinking (Steele & Raider, 2001). Interventions are directed at these experiences and themes within a developmentally appropriate context. The structured drawing activities used in *SITCAP* give children a way to depict their subjective experiences while teaching us what matters most to them in their subjective worlds. Chapter 4 is dedicated entirely to this structured process.

Concept Two: Nonlanguage Activities

Concept two is using nonlanguage activities to help children convey the way they now see themselves, others, and us as a result of their past exposures, as well as using these nonlanguage activities to reconstruct a view that assists in diminishing the survival-driven behaviors associated with trauma.

Remember that in implicit memory, traumatic memories are stored through our senses—what we see, hear, smell, touch, and taste (Rothschild, 2000). These memories are contained in "iconic symbols" (Michaesu & Baettig, 1996). *Iconic symbolization* is the process of giving our experiences a visual identity. Images are created to contain all of the elements of that experience—what happened, our emotional reactions to it, the horror-filled details, and the terror experienced. The trauma experience, therefore, is more easily communicated through imagery. "When a terrifying incident such as trauma is experienced and does not fit into a contextual memory, a new memory is established" (van der Kolk et al., 1996, p. 289). Stated differently, "When memory cannot be linked linguistically, in a contextual framework, it remains at a symbolic level and therefore there are no words to describe it. To retrieve that memory it must be externalized in its symbolic, perceptual iconic form" (Steele, 2003, p. 142).

In order to access this experience, what matters most is that we use sensory-based interventions, such as drawing, that allow children to actually make us a witness to their experiences, to present us with their iconic representations, to give us the opportunity to see what they now see as they look at themselves and the world around them following their exposure to traumatic experiences. In this sense, a picture is worth a thousand words, as shown in the Figure 1.1 drawing by an adolescent who was sexually abused multiple times.

Survival behaviors are formed, driven, and repeated because of how children experienced past traumatic situations and how they are experiencing their current situation, environment, and people in their environment. When they feel unsafe, threatened, or powerless, trauma-related survival behaviors emerge. When children are direct victims of repeated trauma, such as abuse, or exposed to multiple traumas, survival behaviors become more acute and include primitive, survival-directed fight, flight, and freeze behaviors, such as the following:

- ➤ **Fight behaviors** can include verbal attacks, aggressiveness, assaultive behavior, and defiance.
- ➤ **Flight responses** can include running away, refusal to talk, avoiding previous relationships and activities, dissociation, numbing out, substance usage and abuse, eating-disordered behaviors, depression, becoming suicidal, and engaging in other at-risk behaviors.
- ➤ **Freeze responses** can include being unable to make decisions or care for oneself, being lethargic, being nonresponsive, and being unable to interact or sustain relationships.

It makes sense from this perspective that when traumatized children are able to experience themselves, others, and the world, not as victims but as survivors, these

Figure 1.1   Sexual abuse

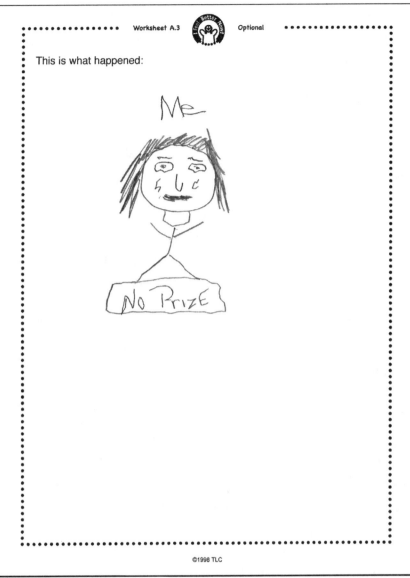

Worksheet A.3   Optional

This is what happened:

©1998 TLC

behaviors decrease. Such behaviors are difficult to diminish through talk-based therapies because they are driven by the way children are experiencing themselves and their worlds, not by higher-level thinking and problem solving. When we help children experience themselves differently, new behaviors emerge, as the practice outcomes and evidence-based research of *SITCAP* has demonstrated.

Concept Three: Using Trauma-Specific Questions

Concept three is using structured, trauma-specific questions to help children tell their story in ways that describe how they are experiencing each of the 10 major themes or subjective experiences addressed in the *SITCAP* model, such as feeling unsafe, powerless, and worried. These and their associated activities are described throughout the text.

The trauma-specific questions incorporated into the sensory process are very structured in order to address the major experience of the session being utilized, for example, the experience of hurt. The questions are not leading and do not ask about feelings, but they are in response to details given by the child. For example, if the child's response to the question "Where do you feel the hurt the most in your body?" is "in my stomach," then the follow-up question might be, "And what happens to your stomach when the hurt is at its worst?" This might be followed by, "Who or what makes the hurt go away?" These questions allow the intervener to remain curious and interesting to the child. At the same time, they help children work within a contained framework to safely elaborate the details of their memories and their experiences, to put their memories into a contextual framework. Once in a contextual framework, it becomes easier for children to begin to cognitively reframe their experiences in ways they can now manage. The specific questions and associated process are discussed in Chapter 5.

Concept Four: Being Curious

Concept four is remaining curious rather than analytical, following children's lead, and avoiding all interpretations, judgments, and assumptions about what they may need.

Children feel most comfortable when we take an interest in their worlds, when we are listening close enough to remain curious about what they tell us without being judgmental, interpreting their comments, or making assumptions. This is generally not an easy process initially for many professionals who were trained to be analytical, to think ahead, and to try to figure out the meaning of the information given by the child.

In TLC's certification training for Trauma and Loss Specialist, it generally takes two days of active participation for practitioners to become comfortable with being curious and imaginative rather than being in the "why?" mindset, which actually prohibits us from being attentive to children. For example, one child who saw his father kill his mother and was later kidnapped by his father only to witness further violence by his father and be left alone for long periods in a grungy room was asked, "What in that room let you feel the safest?" His response was "the couch." When we present this story in our training and then ask the participants what they would ask next, those who have not yet switched to being curious find it difficult to answer because they are too busy trying to figure out the meaning for themselves. Those who, at this point in the training, are able to be curious are quite spontaneous. In essence they follow up immediately with the question, "What about the couch made you feel safe?" Learning how to become a witness—curious rather than analytical—is important to the child's sense of safety and comfort with us and to the success of the intervention process. Being curious rather than analytical is addressed in greater detail in Chapter 5.

Concept Five: Safely Beginning and Ending

Concept five is beginning and ending each session in a safe place with interactions or activities children acknowledge are safe, comforting, and enjoyable.

Self-regulation, the ability to regulate one's reactions to stressful events and threatening situations, is a key component of trauma-informed practice (Hill & Updegraff, 2012; Linehan, Bohus, & Lynch, 2010). Self-regulation refers to the body-mind connection and the ability to use the body as a resource in healing. Stien and Kendall (2004) recommend that the body be used to involve new implicit memories in direct contrast to the traumatic experiences of the past.

> In work with chronically traumatized children in a residential setting, Ziegler (2002) finds that these individuals present with persistently activated arousal. By teaching the children to raise and lower arousal levels by inducing arousal reactions and then returning to a calm state, the children learned what to do with their bodies when faced with a threatening situation, and in so doing Ziegler notes that children became much better at self-regulation. (Steele & Malchiodi, 2012, p. 77)

When practitioners help children become aware of their sensory experiences, an integrated healing process begins. During the intervention process, we want to help children experience a sense of safety, a sense of calmness in their body before and following attention given to traumatic experiences. In essence, we want them to arrive at the conviction that "Even though my memories sometimes scare me and upset me, I will be okay because I can calm myself or deactivate activated reactions triggered by trauma memories" (Langmuir, Kirsch, & Classen, 2012). This concept is further discussed in Chapter 3.

By beginning and ending in a safe place and attending to the trauma work in between, we are containing the trauma in a way that helps children remain safe but also gives them the opportunity to engage in activities that reinforce their ability to go to that safe place and regulate their responses when they are fearful.

Concept Six: Reframing the Experience

Concept six is delaying cognitive reframing until children reveal how they are now making sense of what they are experiencing as a result of the intervention.

Attempting to use language to help traumatized children heal while their predominant responses to daily life are from the midbrain, limbic region has very limited success. For children to accept our efforts to help cognitively reframe their experience and their view of self and others in ways they can now better manage, they must first experience that cognitive explanation at a sensory level. Cognitive reframing is important to healing

Figure 1.2   Trauma is only one part of my life

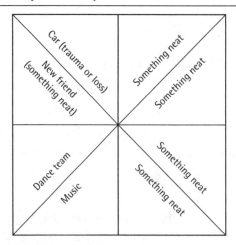

and is integrated into *SITCAP*, but only after being with children in sensory activities designed to support the desired cognitive explanations. Its use is discussed at length in Chapter 5; following is one example.

Using Figure 1.2 as a reference, create eight sections on a plain piece of paper. Now, going back in time, select one loss or trauma experience that is personal to you. Select a word or phrase that identifies that experience for you. If this experience was related to a car fatality, the word "car" might reflect that experience. Now write that word in one of the eight sections. Next, think about some of the fun, exciting, or interesting things that have happened in your life, and using the same process, select a word that reflects each of those experiences and write it in each of the remaining seven sections—put one fun experience in each section. It is sometimes helpful to provide simple examples, such as learning to ride a bike, some fun event at school, a friend, being on the dance team, or a vacation.

Now, as you look at the sections on your paper, what statement about you and trauma jumps out at you? The general response to this activity is that "Life is more than just trauma" or "Trauma is just one part of my life. There are many different parts of my life that make me who I am." This is a very simple activity and one we present in a variety of forms because it sets the foundation for moving from victim thinking to survivor thinking.

However, imagine a teen, whom we will call Martha, is in need of your help. Martha has experienced a horrible trauma, and you attempt to help her reframe her experience at a cognitive level without engaging in an activity that would help her arrive at this reframing by herself. For example, "Martha, what you've gone through is just horrific. I can't imagine what it has all been like for you, but what I need for you to understand and appreciate, Martha, is that this horrible incident is only one part of who you are. There are many parts, many facets of you—the many things about you that make you who you are today. Trauma does not change that about you."

Now how do you think your verbal effort is going to be experienced by Martha? When we present this verbal response in training, participants feel like we are minimizing her experience and, in so many words, saying "get over it." However, if you take Martha through the above activity, she will arrive at that conclusion for herself. Now your effort at reframing what she has arrived at through this sensory activity can be more easily accepted and integrated into her view of self. Cognitive reframing is very important to healing, but the reframing must reflect what has been experienced at a sensory level. Additional examples of the reframing process specific to the sensory experience are presented in Chapter 6.

Practice–Based Evidence (PBE) and Evidence–Based Practice (EBP) Outcomes

In this section we identify the essential research criteria needed to support an intervention's value. Although somewhat detailed, we find that an intervention will more likely be pursued and trusted when the criteria supporting its value are identified. The criteria address those interventions that have years of practiced history and documented, positive outcomes and those whose outcomes are the result of formal evidence-based research. *SITCAP* meets the criteria for both formal research and practice history.

It makes sense that an intervention be selected based on documented, desirable outcomes appropriate to the unique needs and characteristics of the population it is intended to help. Kasdin (2000) reviewed the existence of available intervention programs discussed in the literature. He identified 500 such interventions, but fewer than 10% had undergone any experimental research. For this reason, "The Society for the School of Psychology and various divisions in the American Psychological Association began developing mechanisms for validating interventions as evidence based in the mid-1990s" (Dietrich, 2008).

Dietrich (2008) suggests that an intervention that has a history of producing repetitive, documented desired outcomes is evidence of the value of that practice. Evidence-based practice, on the other hand, requires that desirable outcomes be reported by at least one empirically controlled study (APA, Presidential Task Force on Evidence-Based Practice, 2005). Today there still remains a great deal of discussion and varied differences in interpretation as to what constitutes practice-based evidence (PBE) and evidence-based practice (EBP). To avoid getting lost in the maze of researcher questions, challenges, and differences surrounding what constitutes valid evidence today, we present the following elements of an intervention that we believe make it of value to the practitioner and those children that intervention is intended to help:

> ➤ The intervention has proven useful in multiple settings with diverse cultures.
> ➤ The intervention has demonstrated, in varied settings such as schools and clinical settings, consistent documented outcomes over time (minimum of 10 years) with

varied treatment populations, such as children victimized by violent incidents as well as those exposed to nonviolent grief-inducing incidents.

➤ The intervention is practical, meaning it can be used by most practitioners as a group or individual process and is fairly easy to learn.

➤ The intervention is manualized to allow for greater practice fidelity so it can be accurately evaluated and appropriately used.

➤ The intervention has undergone at least one controlled empirical research study using an evidence-based research model, and has documented significant reduction of symptoms, in this case PTSD and related mental health symptoms.

➤ The intervention is based on well-researched, articulated findings involving neuroscience, resilience, and strength-based research.

➤ The intervention process is well accepted and supported by practitioners of various disciplines and by varied populations.

➤ The intervention lends itself to ongoing evaluation in multiple settings with diverse populations.

The *SITCAP* model meets all of these criteria. The model includes the following programs: *I Feel Better Now!* and *Structured Sensory Interventions for Traumatized At-Risk and Adjudicated Adolescents and Adults*. These programs cover children and adolescents from ages 6 through 18 and are designed for both group and individual intervention. Rather than providing a detailed statistical summary of their research history, which can be found in published studies (Raider & Steele, 2010; Steele, Kuban, & Raider, 2009; Steele & Raider, 2001; Steele, Raider, Delillo-Storey, Jacobs, & Kuban, 2008), we present a brief summary that supports the value of these programs based on the suggested criteria associated with PBE and EBP.

The *I Feel Better Now!* program was first field-tested in 1993 in 13 school districts and at three community agencies. A total of 150 children ages 6 to 12 completed this eight-session, sensory-based group intervention. The outcomes showed that 100% of the parents and each of the 80 practitioners providing the intervention recommended the program and saw significant changes in the children's behavior, even though the program did not focus on behavior but rather the subjective experiences induced by the children's grief and/or trauma exposures. Children were exposed to both violent and nonviolent situations, and the majority had multiple exposures.

In 2007 through 2008, *I Feel Better Now!* underwent additional formal evidence-based research involving 100 children in three different schools. Three standard assessment tools were used to evaluate outcomes between the treatment groups and waitlist groups, all groups at the beginning and end of the intervention program, and three months and six months later with no additional intervention. The Briere Trauma Symptom Checklist (Briere, 1966), the Achenbach Child Behavior Checklist (Achenbach and Rescorla, 2001), and the PTSD Child Questionnaire (Steele et al., 2009) all indicated statistically significant

Table 1.1   *I Feel Better Now!* Program Outcomes

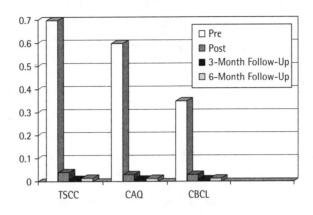

Table 1.2   At–Risk Adjudicated Adolescent Outcomes

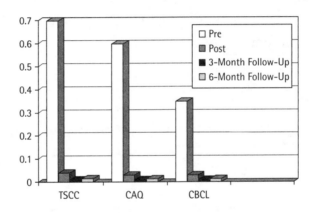

reduction of PTSD and related mental health reactions at the end of intervention and at three and six months following the end of intervention, as illustrated in Table 1.1.

From 2006 through 2007, the adolescent program *Structured Sensory Intervention for At-Risk and Adjudicated Adolescents* underwent formal evidence-based research with at-risk and adjudicated adolescents in a residential setting. The same three standardized evaluation tools (adolescent versions) used to evaluate the *I Feel Better Now!* program were used in this controlled evidence-based research.

Table 1.2 presents the outcome of this evidence-based study. It demonstrates significant reductions in trauma-related and mental health–related symptoms at the end of intervention and three months following the last intervention. In addition, significant reductions were seen in anxiety, thought and attention problems, rule-breaking and aggressive behaviors, and internalizing and externalizing behaviors. Earlier studies by others of cognitive-behavioral interventions (Ovaert, Cashel, & Sewell, 2003) with adjudicated adolescents did not demonstrate reduction in symptoms of anxiety, anger, and depression. It can be hypothesized that the combination of sensory interventions followed by cognitive interventions produced additional outcomes. Unique to this research was the use of an intervention Fidelity of Treatment Checklist completed for each participant. Results indicated 98.5% fidelity with the manualized treatment model.

Case Studies

In the two cases cited in Tables 1.3 through 1.6, the Youth Self-Report (Achenbach & Rescorla, 2010) and the Briere Trauma Symptom Child Checklist (Briere, 1996) were used to evaluate for PTSD and related clinically significant mental health symptoms prior to intervention, at the end of intervention (10 sessions), and again in three months. The following two cases illustrate the value of *SITCAP* for children and adolescents who are witnesses to violent, trauma-inducing incidents and for those who are the direct victims of traumatic experiences. Although these cases are specific to violence, the more detailed published outcomes of *SITCAP* research (Steele et al., 2008) show statistically significant reduction of symptoms in children exposed to single and multiple nonviolent and violent losses and trauma.

Repeated Abuse

Tables 1.3 and 1.4 show the significant reduction of trauma and mental health–related symptoms of 15-year-old Ruy who, over a long period of time had been abused,

Table 1.3   Case "R": Pre vs. Post Briere Trauma Symptom Checklist (TSCC-A)

Briere TSCC-A Scores	PRE	POST	3-MONTH*
Anxiety	9	2	1
Depression	14	3	3
Anger	22	5	4
Posttraumatic Stress	15	4	3
Dissociation	18	5	1

*3-month follow-up post-intervention

Table 1.4   Case "R": Pre vs. Post Achenbach Youth Self-Report (YSR)

Achenbach YSR Scores	PRE	POST	3-MONTH*
Attention Problems	8	4	4
Rule-Breaking Behavior	13	9	2
Aggression	13	11	3
Internalizing Behavior	15	4	3
Externalizing Behavior	26	10	1
Total Problems	63	23	20

*3-month follow-up post-intervention

Table 1.5 Case "S": Pre vs. Post Briere Trauma Symptom Checklist (TSCC-A)

Briere TSCC-A Scores	PRE	POST	3-MONTH*
Anger	9	2	2
Posttraumatic Stress	9	5	3
Dissociation	10	1	1

*3-month follow-up post-intervention

Table 1.6 Case "S": Pre vs. Post Achenbach Youth Self–Report (YSR)

Achenbach YSR Scores	PRE	POST	3-MONTH*
Social Problems	7	0	3
Thought Problems	12	6	2
Attention Problems	12	3	2
Aggression	12	2	2
Internalizing Problems	16	2	1
Externalizing Problems	18	9	1
Total Problems	73	23	20

*3-month follow-up post-intervention

neglected, and repeatedly raped before being removed from her drug-addicted parents. Although additional intervention was needed to especially assist her with socialization and developing relationships, posttraumatic growth became much easier with the reduction of PTSD and related mental health symptoms realized by engaging her in the sensory experiences of *SITCAP*.

Witness to Domestic Violence

Tables 1.5 and 1.6 show the significant gains made by Steve, a 12-year-old boy who witnessed the repeated abuse of his mother by his father and later his stepfather. Always living in fear of the next beating, Steve developed several trauma-specific and mental health–related symptoms, as shown in the above tables. He was failing in school and constantly fighting. By introducing him to new experiences via the *SITCAP* intervention, his view of self, others, and life changed, and his trauma-related behaviors diminished significantly.

Summary

The 23 years of practice- and evidence-based research supports the value of *SITCAP*. What makes this set of programs unique is its focus on attending to how children are experiencing their life, the use of structured sensory activities to reduce PTSD and related mental health reactions, its use with violent and nonviolent grief- and trauma-inducing experiences, and its use in multiple settings with diverse populations. We introduced this chapter with the mandate from grieving and traumatized children, and discussed that what matters most are not their symptoms but how children are experiencing them-selves, others, and life as a result of exposure to grief and/or trauma-inducing incidents.

This approach is such an essential part of the *SITCAP* process that in Chapter 2 we expand on its importance to children and practitioners. We present Alicia's story to illustrate that a diagnosis does not necessarily tell us what is going to matter the most in our efforts to help children. After describing some of the differences between grief and trauma, we examine how children's experiences shape their private logic and their thoughts about self and others, and how these induce trauma-driven, survival behaviors. The chapter then concludes with the rationale for incorporating sensory-based experi-ences into the *SITCAP* programs.

CHAPTER TWO

Children's Experiences With Grief and Trauma

This chapter elaborates on why approaching grief and trauma as an experience rather than as a diagnostic category is critical to avoiding erroneous assumptions as to what children are experiencing, preventing the possibility of "overintervening," and determining what matters most to children's efforts to manage their reactions. It discusses the role that safety and *private logic* have in shaping and driving survival behavior and what is needed to alter these behaviors, which can be very challenging to others and frustrating and troublesome for the children. We expand on the reason why talk therapy and cognitive-based interventions are initially of limited assistance in our initial efforts to help and, as is detailed in subsequent chapters, are most effective when preceded by sensory-based intervention. We conclude with a case example that illustrates that symptoms alone do not reveal what really matters most to grieving and traumatized children.

Before we get started, we want to present you with a few questions. The first two questions are related to our discussion regarding the primary experience of and difference between grief and trauma. We then ask you to identify the one statement, among several related grief statements, that reflects a trauma-related reaction. The final task is to complete the incomplete sentences we present, which reflect the private logic of severely traumatized children. The answers are presented sequentially in this chapter.

The first two questions:

1. What one word can we use to describe the overall experience of grief? When we say, for example, that someone is grieving, we say they are usually feeling what?
2. What one word can we then use that would best describe the experience of trauma?

The following statements are from children whose siblings were dying from cancer or who had died recently. After each statement, ask yourself whether the statement reflects a grief response, a trauma response, or both grief and trauma. If you indicate that a reaction represents both grief and trauma, we would then ask you what factors would distinguish one from the other.

➤ (Describing a dream) "My sister is falling through a dimension and there are bad guys chasing and shooting at her."
➤ "Sometimes I think I caused it; like it was my fault."

➤ "I get jealous sometimes because my brother gets all the attention and sometimes I do mean things like break some of his stuff."

➤ "I don't want to talk about it."

This final task is related to private logic and its role in shaping behavior. We present several incomplete sentences that we want you to try to complete. Later in the chapter you can compare your responses to ours.

➤ I must do something to let you know . . .

➤ I will do whatever I need to do in order to . . .

➤ I will fight any experience, any activity, or any person that tries to control me because . . .

➤ I will not do what you want me to do because if I do and . . .

Subjective Experiences of Grief and Trauma

Table 2.1 illustrates a few of the differences between a grief and a trauma experience. Each is discussed in the following pages.

Table 2.1   Differences Between Grief and Trauma

Grief	Trauma
Generalized reaction: SADNESS	Generalized reaction: TERROR
Grief reactions can stand alone.	Trauma reactions generally also include grief reactions.
Grief reactions are generally known to the public and the professional.	Trauma reactions, especially in children, are largely unknown to the public and often to professionals.
In grief, guilt says, "I wish I would or would not have . . . "	Trauma guilt says, "It was my fault. I could have prevented it. It should have been me."
Grief generally does not attack or "disfigure" our identity.	Trauma generally attacks, distorts, and "disfigures" our identity.
In grief, dreams tend to be of the person who died.	In trauma, dreams are about the child him- or herself dying or being hurt.
In grief, pain is related to the loss.	In trauma, pain is related to the tremendous terror and an overwhelming sense of powerlessness and fear for safety.
In grief, a child's anger is generally not destructive.	In trauma, a child's anger often becomes assaultive (even after nonviolent trauma, fighting often increases).

Trauma reactions are DIFFERENT from grief reactions
Trauma reactions OVERPOWER grief reactions

Children can be traumatized by violent or nonviolent incidents. Separation from a parent through divorce or foster care, a family member's terminal illness or sudden death, exposure to physical or sexual abuse, witness of drug use, surviving a house fire, experiencing extreme weather such as tornados, floods, earthquakes, or hurricanes, as well as witnessing drowning, murder, suicide, and school violence can all be traumatizing incidents.

When we say someone is experiencing grief, the one word that best describes that experience is *sadness*. If sadness is the primary experience, then having the time to simply be sad while receiving comfort and assistance in meeting basic needs will be helpful. When we say someone is experiencing trauma, the one word that best describes that experience is *terror*. We define *terror* as feeling totally unsafe and powerless to do anything about one's situation (Steele, 2003). If the primary experience of trauma is feeling unsafe and powerless, it makes sense that interventions should be directed at restoring that sense of safety and power. Because trauma involves many losses, our efforts to help must also address the grief reactions that may have resulted from trauma. However, someone who is grieving may only be grieving. In other words, trauma can include the reactions of grief, but grief can stand alone. We note here that, although we are identifying several distinct differences between grief and trauma, the reality is that at times we simply cannot be sure whether a child is grieving or in trauma. We developed *SITCAP (Structured Sensory Interventions for Traumatized Children, Adolescents and Parents)* as an intervention that would address both experiences while also assisting in the identification of those clinically significant subjective experiences needing attention.

Keep in mind our discussion in Chapter 1 indicating that trauma is not a cognitive experience, but an *implicit*, sensory experience. This means trying to verbally reassure terrified children that they are safe will generally have little impact; they have to experience that sense of safety for themselves. Also keep in mind that in the *implicit* world, sensations and feelings are the dominant conveyers that determine how we feel and ultimately how we act. If we are sensing some threat, even if it is not real, our body and brain prepares itself to survive; our entire being moves into a state of readiness. It will take some other nonthreatening sensory experience to calm and deactivate our heightened state of readiness. Explained in a different way, ask yourself: "What do mashed potatoes have to do with trauma?"

What Do Mashed Potatoes Have To Do With Trauma?

Approximately three months following 9/11, New Yorkers were understandably still struggling with all they experienced on that terror-filled day. Even though it was months later, people were still seeking help, asking for medications to help them sleep, to calm their anxiety and worries, and to help with their grief as well as trauma. Reassurances of safety were frequently coming from the Oval Office and local government officials, yet these cognitive reassurances were of limited help for many people. What was more helpful? What mattered the most? About three months after 9/11, a survey of New York area restaurants discovered that the consumption of mashed potatoes had tripled since 9/11. What mattered the most was not reason, not logic, but a sensory intervention that calmed their implicit, sensory memories—in this case, comfort food.

Although we do not have a formal reference for the aforementioned survey, we do have a very reputable reference related to efforts to deal with the major financial losses many Americans suffered in Fall 2008 when the stock market plummeted and took with it the dreams of many. Those of us who had saved for years to retire were now hit with the reality that it would take years to recover what was lost in the market that day; retirement would have to wait. It was far too overwhelming to think away the tremendous stress this created in our lives. On September 30, 2008, the *Wall Street Journal* reported the following:

> The defeat of the proposed $700 billion bailout . . . sent U.S. stocks plunging Monday . . . the broad Standard and Poor's 500 had its biggest percentage drop since 1987. The only stock that finished higher from the Standard & Poor's 500 was comfort-food processor Campbell Soup. The title of this article was taken from a statement by Campbell's soup spokesman talking about Campbell's secret to success: "We want comfort when stressed." (Looks like another Black Monday, 2008, p. 6)

Relief Through Sensory Regression

We established in Chapter 1 that when people are extremely stressed, it is difficult to think, much less try to problem solve or even hear what others might be saying. Think about the last time you were really stressed. When you finally got home at the end of the day, you did not sit down and say to yourself, "I am going to talk my way out of this stress." What you probably did was actually regress and engage in some sensory behavior that in the past brought you a sense of comfort and control. For some it's comfort food, for others it might be adding extra time for jogging, reading, or listening to music. The fact is that we can actually regain a sense of calm, comfort, and control over our own reactions by engaging in some (sensory) activity that has brought us this sense of calm in the past, and then we begin to engage in cognitive processes that allow us to problem solve how we are going to manage who or what caused our stress.

When interviewed following 9/11, many educators said that after a few days they couldn't talk about what they had experienced. When asked what was most helpful to them, they shared with us that many of the health clubs opened their doors to educators so they could use the pools and the hot tubs and receive massages. They indicated that this helped them much more than talking. The New York school system, like many large city school systems, is somewhat a bureaucratic system. That day educators had to make several quick and critical decisions on their own because communication with administrators was shut down. Amazingly, they evacuated every child safely, but many students and staff were direct witnesses to all that happened that day. They had very high levels of exposure to the sights, sounds, smells, the taste of pollutants, and the chaos.

After the first few days, they reported that talking only intensified the primary reactions they first experienced that tragic day. Instead, comfort foods like mashed potatoes and soup and other sensory experiences like music and exercise helped the most. The same comfort that is helpful in trauma is helpful in grief, yet the differences between the two experiences are important to identify.

The Differences Matter

Why is it important to understand the differences between grief and trauma? When we understand the differences we can address the differences with children, normalize those reactions, and be less likely to misinterpret their behaviors and apply inappropriate interventions. When a child is stuck in trauma, he continues to react, even months later, as if the danger was still very real. When experiencing life as threatening, it is very difficult to allow ourselves to be sad, because it would leave us feeling far too vulnerable. What we need to feel is safe and empowered. If we do not recognize that a child is in trauma and we attempt to address only his grief, he is likely to resist our efforts, be nonresponsive, or let us know in some way that we are not helping. We review the differences between grief and trauma by examining the children's statements presented at the beginning of the chapter.

"She Is Falling Through a Dimension"

As much anxiety as this dream might cause children, it would be considered a grief-driven dream. In a grief-driven dream, the dreamer is dreaming about something happening to someone else. The dreamer is outside of his dream looking in as an observer. In a trauma-driven dream, the major difference is that the dreamer is actually in his own dream as a potential victim and in potential harm's way. One way to quickly establish the possibility that trauma has been experienced by children is to ask them about their scariest dreams. If they are part of that scary dream, not an outside observer, but in their own dream in potential harm's way, the situation they were exposed to likely induced a trauma-related reaction. So even though in our example, our child, who was dreaming about his sister falling through a dimension and being chased and shot at, is certainly frightened by his dream, he is not likely to experience the kind of terror that he would experience if in fact he were the one who was being chased, shot at, and in potential harm's way.

"So I Broke Some of His Things"

Although the difference between grief and trauma can be difficult to identify, we consider this to be a grief-driven response. This child indicated that he became jealous over all the attention that his dying brother received. When that jealousy went unattended, he needed to find some way to more effectively communicate his need for some attending—in this case, breaking some of his brother's things. Grief-driven anger is generally oppositional; in other words, you'll hear "no," "I'm not going to," "You can't make me," and other defiant reactions. In trauma-driven anger, the dynamic is different. Ask yourself, "What are the rewards for fighting?" The common responses we receive when we pose this question in our trainings are that fighting releases the stress and tension in the body that is created when we become angry, brings attention to us, and most importantly brings us a sense of power.

In grief-driven anger, we are not stripped of our sense of power. At the core of trauma is an overwhelming sense of powerlessness—the inability to do anything about what is happening. In trauma-driven anger, we often see an increase in aggressive and assaultive, rule-breaking behavior, especially at those times when trauma memories have been activated. This trauma-driven, rule-breaking behavior and fighting response often happens without warning, is directed at whomever happens to be around at the time, and often occurs for no apparent reason. In grief, if there is fighting, that fighting is generally directed at a sibling or a very good friend.

The prescription for grief-driven anger is to provide the attention children often need by spending time with them. The fighting response of trauma becomes more critical, because it puts everyone involved at greater physical and emotional risk. Human nature drives us to free ourselves of fear and anxiety. We will repeat any behavior that reduces our fears, even when that behavior is self-defeating or self-destructive. If fighting restores our sense of power, then we will repeat the behavior when feeling powerless or unsafe, as is often seen with traumatized children. The prescription for trauma-driven anger is to engage children in sensory activities that allow them to experience a sense of power in ways that are not self-defeating or hurtful to self or others, which we accomplish in the *SITCAP* program, as demonstrated by the research presented in Chapter 1.

"It Was My Fault"

This response could be a grief- or trauma-driven response. We would need to know if the child is experiencing additional layers of guilt associated with trauma-driven guilt. How is grief-driven guilt different from trauma-driven guilt? In grief-driven guilt, especially with younger children, we often hear magical thinking. Sometimes simply saying to children there is nothing they could do, think, say, or wish that could have caused this to happen will be all children need to hear in order to feel better. However, keep in mind that this is a cognitive intervention. If the child in our example was also traumatized by that death, then it's very likely that this cognitive intervention would not be helpful. We would need to involve that child in a sensory intervention that would allow him to arrive at the conclusion that he doesn't have those kinds of magical powers. A simple example might be saying to the child, while you're sitting together, "I'm going to count to three, and as I'm counting to three, I want you to get all your magical powers ready to go, so when I reach three you can use your magical powers and [for example, if there is a television in the room] turn the television on without using the remote." Obviously we select a simple challenge. Following the failure of his magical powers, when we now say, "You see, there is nothing you could think or wish or do that could cause your grandpa to die," he is more likely to be able to understand and accept the concept. This, of course, needs to be balanced by empowering children with the positive ways they can remember their loved ones.

It is interesting to note that many of the reactions we apply to grieving children are also experienced by adults. Magical thinking is one of these reactions. In the early 1990s, when working with adult survivors of homicide, hearing adult survivors describe magical thinking was not unusual. One mother's son was shot in a "drive-by" outside of her home. She heard the shot and said she knew instantly that her son had been shot. She ran outside to where he was lying on the ground, but she said, "I was afraid to touch him because if I touched him, he would die." This was not an unusual response at such a personally tragic time. Unfortunately, two years later, these responses were causing her tremendous guilt.

Additional Trauma-Driven Guilt Factors

Why Not Me?

In trauma-driven guilt, there are additional factors. Those factors include the thoughts, "Why did I survive? Why did my best friend die and I'm still here?" To determine whether children might be dealing with trauma-driven guilt, one question we can ask is, "Do you sometimes think or wish that it should have been you instead?" When there is a positive response to this question, it's very likely they are experiencing trauma-driven guilt. Trauma guilt is also induced or is caused by additional reactions, such as what we did or did not do to escape, or what we did or did not do to help the victim. Generally, these reactions are not part of the grief response. If they are, it is likely that grief is part of a larger trauma response to what happened.

Poor Judgment/Careless Behavior

There are those cases when guilt is the result of poor judgment or careless behavior. Depending on the outcome, grief may remain the primary experience. However, all too often, situations involving poor judgment or careless behavior are also traumatic. One example is the accidental shooting of a friend or sibling by a child who was playing with a gun in his home. In these situations, we need to help the child understand that we know this was not his intent. In cases where children are direct witnesses to the outcome of poor judgment or careless behavior, we are likely to have to help them with all the sensory, implicit memories of what they saw happen. When a situation is experienced as traumatic, it is very difficult to avoid thinking about the horrid details of what happened, whereas in grief we generally are not focused on details, but rather the pain of the loss and the sadness of realizing our loved one is gone. If this loss also involves being terrified because of what this loss means regarding living arrangements, for example, then it can also become a traumatic experience.

Healing the Guilt and Shame

Shame is often associated with trauma-driven guilt. This shame is frequently associated with the way the body responded to the trauma it was exposed to at the time. Survivors generally do not tell us what happened with their bodies at that time, so it is important to normalize the physiological responses to extreme terror. It helps to briefly educate trauma victims about the fact that the brain prepares and dictates to our body what it needs to do to survive when faced with a terrifying situation. There is no thinking involved; it becomes primarily a midbrain, limbic response. It also helps to have a picture of the brain when explaining which part of the brain triggers our primal survival responses.

Three weeks or even months following exposure, survivors will let us know that they have not been told about how the brain reacts to extreme stress when they ask, "Why did I do this? Why didn't I . . . ?" One way to respond to this is to simply ask them, "Are you alive right now?" Of course they will say "yes," but they might wonder why you are asking. The helpful response is an explanation such as the following:

> You are alive now because your brain activated your body to do what it needed to do to survive. Your survival brain took over your thinking brain. Now that you're safe and your survival brain is not so activated, your thinking brain is working hard to understand what happened by presenting you with all the should-haves and could-haves of all that might have been different. The fact is that, from a purely neurological perspective, at that point in time, you couldn't think. You really don't need to feel responsible for what happened at that moment in time, because under extreme stress we never know how we are going to respond, even when we are well trained to manage frightening situations.

When we normalize the possible reactions to this nonthinking moment in time, we want to also include the following: "I wouldn't be surprised if you wet yourself, or pooped on yourself, or tried to help but your body would not move, or tried to scream for help but nothing came out." This explanation of the neurology of trauma and normalization of trauma reactions can often bring a great deal of relief to those who were feeling responsible and ashamed because of the way they and their bodies reacted.

At Its Core

The *SITCAP* program focuses not on symptoms such as guilt, but rather on the overall experience. Helping survivors heal from their guilt presents a good example of how focusing on the experience rather than the symptom can lead to symptom reduction. Over the years we have found that guilt is really a response to an underlying feeling that is common to trauma and to sudden and unexpected loss. Many years ago, there was a sniper attack at an elementary school that left several students and staff critically wounded. When Robert Pynoos and his colleagues from the University of California at Los Angeles (UCLA) evaluated the impact that incident had on the children, they found that the children who were not there at the time of the shooting had a higher level of severity of guilt than the children who were there at the time (Pynoos & Eth, 1986). We have to ask ourselves, "Why would they be experiencing more guilt than the ones who were actually there?" The primary responses of the children who were not there are reflected in these frequent responses to trauma-driven guilt: "If I had been there, I would've been able to do something to prevent my best friend from getting shot" or "If I had been there, it would have been me instead." Essentially, these children were feeling powerless about all that happened in their absence. Our research over the years has shown that when trauma victims are able to regain a sense of safety and empowerment, guilt and other PTSD-related symptoms diminish. The overall *SITCAP* process is designed to restore a sense of empowerment for this reason.

In both grief- and trauma-driven guilt, it is important to normalize the possible reactions, because survivors tend to not talk about their guilt, especially any shame they experience. In both situations there is a sense of feeling powerless that, when restored, significantly reduces the guilt response. However, in trauma-driven guilt there are multiple reactions not generally experienced in grief, such as shame. In these situations, sustaining the sense of empowerment through multiple sensory activities over time is important to healing from trauma-driven guilt.

"I Don't Want to Talk About It"

Is this a grief or trauma response? It could be both; we need to know a little bit more about what that child was experiencing to determine whether this was a grief or trauma response. It could be that he simply was tired of hearing people say that they were sorry or that he wasn't getting the comfort he needed or hearing what he needed to hear at that point in time. If this was his experience, then his response would be more of a grief response. However, we know that how others respond to what happens to us influences our willingness to tell others what we are experiencing.

When children are traumatized, the instinctive response is to want to tell someone about what happened, and that someone is typically the significant adult in their life at the time. When children are given the opportunity to tell their parent(s), for example, about the details of what happened, what often happens to the parent? The parent becomes anxious and unsure of what to say or what to do. A child senses their parent's anxiety, and the anxiety of both the parent and the child increases to a point where that parent may say, "You know, the more we talk about this, the more upset we both get, so let's not talk about it anymore." What unfortunate lesson do children in this interaction learn from this response? They learn that the *big people* in their life cannot manage what they have experienced. Therefore, when they come to our attention and we ask if they'd like to tell us what happened, their initial response is "no." This means that we really have to present ourselves as being curious about what happened and give children the opportunity to communicate to us what their experience was like, often in ways that do not involve language. Asking children to draw a picture of what happened is one way to provide the medium needed to accomplish this. Drawing is one of the primary interventions in the *SITCAP* programs and is discussed in detail in Chapter 4.

A Stuttering-Like Response

We also find at times that children may attempt to tell us what happened, but in the process they begin to have difficulty forming the words, similar to stuttering. The literature shows that stuttering is frequently associated with PTSD (Kates, 2009). Consider for a moment that you've gone through life without any difficulties talking. Then you are exposed to a trauma, and when you go to tell someone about what happened, you find it becomes difficult to get the words out; you experience a stuttering-like response. If this were to happen to you, what one thought might you have in response to your own stuttering? Very likely that thought would be along the lines of "I guess talking about it only makes it worse." If a child has had this response, we can appreciate the fear it would induce and why that child might want to avoid talking about what happened. This is another reason why drawing can be so helpful. Talking is not necessary for children to bring us into their world. However, it is generally easier for children to use their drawings as a *show and tell*, then to simply attempt to answer questions without such a visual reference point. As the anxiety of PTSD is reduced, so too is the stuttering response, unless there is also an indication of social anxiety beyond PTSD, as stuttering is frequently related to social anxiety (Stuttered Speech Syndrome, 2012).

Repressive Coping: Is It Avoidance or Resilience?

The reason why children may not want to talk about their trauma experience may be as simple as not feeling safe enough with us to do so, or that they have discovered that it works better for them not to talk about what happened. Talking is not always the solution. We will find in our discussion on resilience in Chapter 9 that *repressive coping*—the decision to not talk about something unpleasant—is a characteristic of many resilient children. If children are doing well by coping in this manner, we certainly do not want to suggest that they need to talk about something they are managing well, or they will get worse, or possibly become defiant or oppositional in our efforts to help.

If children are not managing well and want to avoid talking about what happened, then their effort to avoid what has been terrifying is not helping.

What makes *SITCAP* unique is that its sensory process can help traumatized children find relief from their experiences without talking about those experiences. However, in some cases, children have no memory of their traumatic past, and yet what their body experiences and their behaviors are the outcome of that trauma. In these cases we simply work with children in the present by asking them, for example, "What is your biggest worry today or this week?" We then follow this with specific sensory activities associated with worry. As their present worry diminishes, the anxiety that has accumulated since their traumatic experience begins to lessen as well. In a sense, worry is worry no matter its source, and no matter whether it began long ago or recently.

Similar to our recent understanding that grief is much more of an individual experience today and that not everyone moves through the same stages, we are now recognizing that some children do better not remembering, not being asked to revisit or talk about what happened. As practitioners we must give children a choice to say, "No. I do not want to talk about it or draw about it." However, we must also be sensitive to the fact that this initial response may be resulting from the way others responded to them in the past. This is why the *SITCAP* process begins with educating and normalizing for children the many possible reactions they may be having because of their experiences. We also educate them about what we will be asking them to do, presenting varied examples of what other children have done and how this has helped those children and could help them. We assure them that we are in fact curious about what their experience was or is like, but that they can say "no" to anything we ask them to do or talk about and that "this is perfectly okay because we have lots of other things we can do." A "no" response following this kind of introduction suggests that it may be safer to focus on how the child is experiencing the present, not the past. In this situation, we would reinforce what is going well and help with what is not going well by using sensory-based interventions when appropriate. Safety is the cornerstone of any trauma-informed practice and is discussed in detail in the next chapter.

"The Sound of My Dog Coming Down the Stairs"

This statement references a trauma-specific response. The child, who indicated that the sound of his dog coming down the stairs reminded him of his daddy falling down the stairs, reflects a trauma memory. The child's response is referred to as a *startle response*. The startle response is related to those sensory conditions, like the sound of his dog coming down the stairs, that existed at the time of the traumatic incident, which when reexperienced tend to take us back to that experience. What made this accident traumatic for this child was that his father died as a result of his fall.

A trauma-specific question we want to ask of any child who we think may have been traumatized is "Are there any sounds that remind you of, any smells that remind you of, anything that you see, anything that you hear that reminds you of what happened [each is asked separately]?" Keep in mind that when our midbrain is aroused, we relate to our environment by paying greater attention to our senses—what we see, what we hear, what we sense is about to happen. If there's a sound that's similar to what we heard when that "bad" thing happened, or a smell, or a visual that is similar to what we saw, our trauma memory is triggered, and then our bodies prepare to engage in survival responses based on what we sense we need to do to protect ourselves, even when that threat is not real. This has great significance for us as helpers.

There are four additional factors to consider in our efforts to help grieving and traumatized children. We now discuss those additional factors and then introduce Alicia's story to begin to illustrate *SITCAP*'s use with grieving children and in subsequent chapters with traumatized children.

Resistance, Safety, Duration, and Children's Iconic Identity

We have established several of the differences between grief and trauma. We established that grief may stand alone, but trauma, and the significant losses associated with it, also induces grief. For this reason, we want a trauma intervention that also assists children with the grief they may experience. *SITCAP* helps diminish these reactions. However, there are several other factors to consider when working with traumatized children. These include the need for safety, the issue of resistance to intervention, the view of self that is often altered by trauma, private logic and its associated survival behaviors, and what a diagnosis does not necessarily reveal.

In Trauma There Is No Such Thing as Resistance

Consider that we may be very skilled clinicians, counselors, or social workers, but maybe our hair is parted on the wrong side, or we conduct ourselves in a certain way, or have a certain tone of voice or way of speaking that reminds a child of that bad person who did that bad thing to him. When this happens, that child cannot feel safe with us. This is why there really is no such thing as *resistance* in treatment when we are dealing with traumatized children; either they feel safe with us or they do not. Again, our primary responsibility is to ensure that children are feeling safe—if not with us, then with one of our colleagues. This really is a good example of the neurological impact of trauma and how once we understand the sensory issues related to trauma, we begin to alter how we relate to and intervene with traumatized children.

Agoraphobia or a Need for Safety?

Following 9/11, several studies indicated that a large number of children were experiencing agoraphobia (Hoven et al., 2005). This research supported the extreme impact this act of terror had on many children. However, if we approach trauma as an experience, we may want to ask whether this was true agoraphobia or agoraphobic-like behavior. For example, what if we were one of the children, as was the case for many in New York that day, who saw people jumping to their death, who were only blocks away and covered in the white dust that covered Ground Zero, who saw others running terrified in the streets, who were being carried to safety by a teacher only to hit a police roadblock and be told that we would have to go back through the same chaotic, terrifying environment in order to get to the available evacuation route: Why, after finally getting home, would we want to go back to that bad place where that bad thing happened? Is our reaction really agoraphobic or simply expressing the need for safety?

Duration

Keep in mind that during the six months after 9/11 there were additional threats (anthrax, for example) and the plane that crashed in the Bronx. These incidents kept everyone vigilant and scared for months. This caused initial reactions to be extended over a longer period than the four-week duration criteria for assigning the diagnosis PTSD as indicated in the *DSM-IV-TR*. (Currently, the duration of symptoms must exist for four weeks from the time of initial exposure to assign PTSD.) Given this example, the new duration criteria of six months recommended by the proposed Developmental Trauma Disorder and now being included in the *DSM-5* (APA, 2012) makes more sense with the real-life experiences of trauma. When we approach trauma as experience, it gives a different meaning to the behavior that we are seeing.

"You're No Prize"

There's one additional critical difference between how we experience ourselves when grieving versus how we experience ourselves in trauma. In grief we do not lose our identity; in trauma our identity is altered and, in extreme cases, completely annihilated. In grief we may worry about who will take care of us and what's going to happen next, but we don't lose the sense of self, the view of self we had prior to the grief experience. It's a different experience with trauma. When we are traumatized, our first common experience is to feel unsafe and powerless—feelings associated with being a victim. Often this victim view of self is short-lived, and in several weeks we reclaim our identity because of the primary support provided that kept us safe and empowered. However, if this view of self as a victim continues, then that experience becomes traumatic for us in that we see ourselves as far more helpless, powerless, unsafe, and vulnerable than we did prior to the experience.

Claudia Jewett-Jarrett wrote *Helping Children Cope with Separation and Loss* (2000). In her book she tells the story of a 4-year-old boy who was adopted. That adoption was a traumatic one for him. Several years later, when he's in one of her groups because of the problems he's been having as a result of that adoption, she becomes quite surprised by his response to the discussion in the group. The group began talking about how babies were born. This child indicated that he wasn't "born that way." Surprised by his response, Jarrett replied, "That's fascinating. You're the first kid I ever met who didn't get born that way. How was it instead?" His response was, "You see what happened was one day my social worker was feeling like having a snack. She opened up a box of Crackerjacks. She looked inside and pulled me out. She said, 'You're no prize' and put me in the trash" (p. 80). This was this child's symbolic image of who he was, his identity.

In the first chapter we indicated that at the sensory level, because there is no language, we develop *iconic symbols* or images that define what that experience was like, that define our reactions to that experience, that define how we now look at ourselves and the world around us as a result of what happened to us. We all know what kind of a child this child became because of the experience that changed his view of self from being of value to being "no prize"—a throwaway child. He obviously became very difficult and very challenging for the people in his life.

We will see in later chapters that in order to alter children's trauma-driven behaviors, we're going to have to alter the way they see themselves and their world. Figures 2.1 and 2.2

Figure 2.1   Nontraumatized child

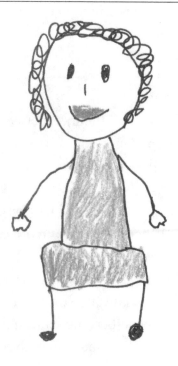

show two self-portraits by children of the same age. (*To protect the confidentiality of children, drawings were reproduced to combine aspects of many children's drawings who were exposed to similar incidents. Case material was also altered to protect the family's identity by including the collective experiences of children exposed to similar experiences. It is also important to note that in the* SITCAP *programs we do not use drawing as an assessment tool, only as a vehicle for children to tell us their stories. Therefore, the only reality as to what children draw in this process is what they tell us the elements of their drawings represent. This will be further discussed in Chapter 4, which is devoted to* SITCAP's *structured drawing process.*)

When we look at Figure 2.1 compared to Figure 2.2, we need to ask "What do each of these identities suggest?" Excluding developmental issues, we are not sure what we are seeing in Figure 2.2, other than it looks distorted. Figure 2.1 actually represents a child who has not experienced any loss or trauma in her life. She is doing quite well, whereas Figure 2.2 is the kind of self-portrait drawn by children who witness the violent beating of others or their own abuse. Looking at this self-portrait, we sense that this child's view of self is likely to result in behaviors that are challenging and perhaps even developmentally delayed. In grief we generally do not see self-portraits that are disfigured, or lack the appropriate (developmental) detail reflected in Figure 2.2, because in grief, our self-identity is not attacked as it is in trauma. The child who witnessed the beating death of her mother describes herself as a weakling, ashamed that she ran into another room while her mother was being beaten and did nothing to help her. What she was exposed to and the understandable actions she took in the face of such terror significantly altered her view of self, which was followed by related

Figure 2.2   Traumatized child

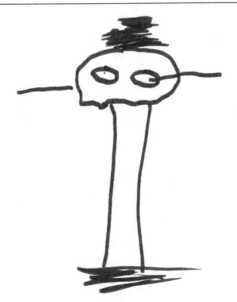

behaviors misdiagnosed as being bipolar by one doctor and reactive attachment disorder by another. Today her behavior, if viewed from a trauma-informed perspective, would be seen as trauma related.

Alicia: What Matters Most

Whether a child is experiencing grief or trauma, the following example supports that symptoms or having a diagnosis do not necessarily tell us what will matter the most to that child's efforts to recover. How children are experiencing what happened to them, and how they see themselves and their world as a result of what happened to them, often provide a better opportunity to discover what matters most to the child. Alicia, an only child, was 8 years old when her mother died of cancer. Her mother spent the last six months of her life moving through the dying process while at home. Alicia was exposed to the many sensory factors associated with dying from a terminal illness, the confusion, the smells, the accidents, the sad, often-difficult-to-look-at withering body of her loved one. Depression, withdrawal, doing poorly in school, and feeling sick, often with no medical cause, are not uncommon in children in this situation. Because she was not creating a behavior problem in the classroom or at home, her call for help was not recognized until one year later.

Using the Child Adolescent Questionnaire (CAQ) to evaluate possible reactions, results indicated moderate to severe avoidant reactions, such as playing with friends less, liking school less, engaging in regressive behaviors, and experiencing somatic reactions. Given that her father worked long hours to support them, her reactions were understandable. The sense was that her grieving had been delayed or stalled, but it was unclear what had or was interrupting this process. For this reason, practitioners are encouraged to give children the opportunity to address every possible subjective experience covered in the *SITCAP* program: fear, terror, worry, anger, hurt, guilt, feeling unsafe, and powerlessness.

After spending time introducing Alicia to what we would be asking her to do, how she could say *yes* or *no*, presenting her with sample drawings of what other children had done, and normalizing her reactions, she was asked to draw a picture of herself. Afterward we talked about what she liked and what she remembered the most about her mother and the fun they had together.

Figure 2.3 is a picture of her sick mother. Taking the position that in this process a drawing only represents what the child tells us it represents, we make no assumptions but become very curious about all the details in that drawing. Pointing to the dots of what looked like her mother's pajama top, Alicia indicated that these were her mother's bad cancer cells. The fact is we never know what we are looking at until the child tells us. Later she drew a picture of her mother on the day she died, represented in Figure 2.4.

Figure 2.3   Sick mother

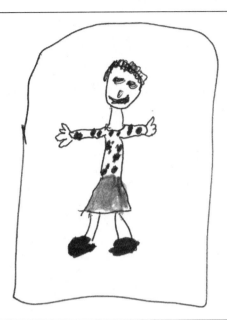

Figure 2.4   Mother deceased

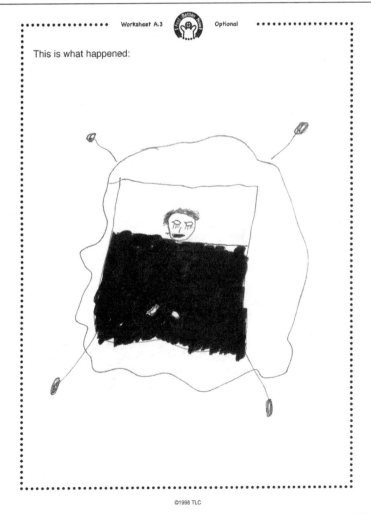

When asked what her biggest worry was since then, she said, "My daddy because he doesn't talk much anymore." She was then asked to color the fish that showed how small or big her worry was. Figure 2.5 shows this to be a significant worry. Worry is addressed because worry is a natural response to any significant loss or trauma, and it is also a form of anxiety. Anything we can do to reduce worry assists in reducing the overall anxiety experienced in grief and trauma.

In session three she was asked to draw what she would like to see happen to what caused her mother to die. What she drew in Figure 2.6 was the bad cancer cells getting "burnt up in a really big fire."

Figure 2.5   Size of Alicia's worry before intervention

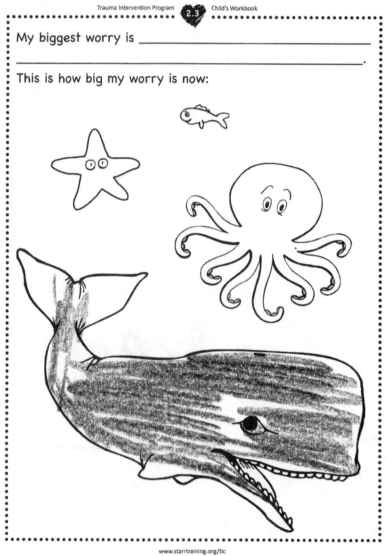

Trauma Intervention Program   **2.3**   Child's Workbook

My biggest worry is _____

_____.

This is how big my worry is now:

www.starrtraining.org/tlc

Figure 2.6   What I would like to see happen to . . .

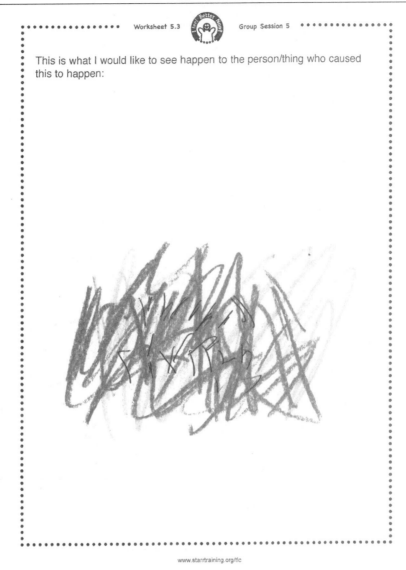

Worksheet 5.3   Group Session 5

This is what I would like to see happen to the person/thing who caused this to happen:

www.starrtraining.org/tlc

This was the turning point for Alicia. From this session on, her father reported that her energy returned. She started talking more often, taking better care of herself, and playing more with her friends. Four weeks later, Alicia's teacher reported that Alicia was doing better with her homework and participating more in class activities. When we asked Alicia in the final session to show us again the size of her worry, Figure 2.7 reflects a major change similar to the reduction of reactions recorded on her CAQ at the end of the program.

Alicia's situation was not as traumatic as the cases we present in subsequent chapters. However, it does help us to appreciate that we can never be sure where children might be

Figure 2.7   Size of Alicia's worry after intervention

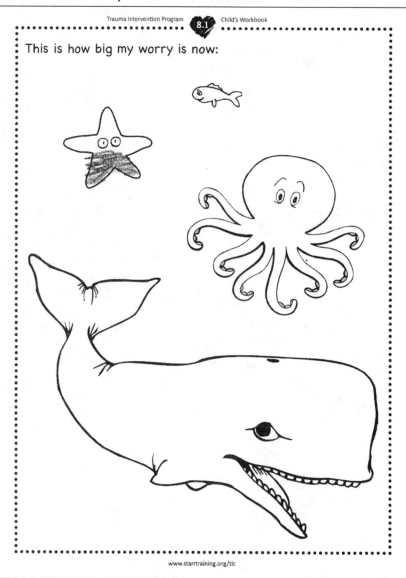

stuck in their experiences, unless we present them with an opportunity to address all the primary experiences of trauma. When we fail to provide children with multiple opportunities to the varied ways that they can experience any grief or trauma situation, our efforts to help may fail to give them an opportunity to find a way to overcome the most difficult part of their experience. For Alicia it was feeling powerless to do anything about those bad cancer cells. Often only one specific aspect of the overall experience triggers the many resulting reactions. Over the years we have often been surprised by what matters most to children, reaffirming that children really are the best experts of what they need to feel better.

Point of Interest

Worry

Recently someone close to me had a medical scare. He was in and out of the emergency room twice in one week. Normally a healthy and active 30-something-year-old, his symptoms were not easy to tolerate or describe. He experienced weakness, fatigue, shallow breathing, and difficulty concentrating. Every test came back normal. Dehydration and possible heat exhaustion were the final diagnoses. Fluids and rest were prescribed. In the weeks that followed, however, his anxiety and overall worry increased. His father died at the age of 42 following a massive heart attack. The anxiety he felt trumped the logic that all of the medical tests came back normal. He is in great physical shape, he exercises regularly, and he does not smoke, but the worry that he may suffer the same fate as his father consumed him.

When the terror of loss of life or safety is presented, you immediately shift away from being able to use the part of your brain that is responsible for reason and logic. It doesn't matter what is said to you by others, even professionals as they attempt to calm your worry. It isn't until you are able to feel safe on a body level that you can begin to believe that you are going to be okay. What my friend knew and understood logically did not matter until his body began to support what others were telling him. He needed to experience not one but several full days doing a variety of activities without symptoms to feel confident about his health again. Remember, it is not what we *say* to others that will lessen worry; it is what we *do* and allow them to experience on a sensory level that matters.

The Private Logic Created by Experiences

In more severe cases, often with histories of multiple exposures, we see very specific changes in children's private logic, which are not generally experienced in grief. It is important to have this discussion because, as we will see, the way we think about ourself, our situation, and others does dictate how we respond to everyday interactions with our environment and the people in the varied environments we must navigate daily. The terror of 9/11, for example, changed how we thought about ourselves as well as how we thought about others. It stripped away our secure sense of safety and our belief that our country was immune from such terror. In the days that followed, we did not think of ourselves as powerful and safe, but as vulnerable. As a result of this one thought, we began to behave differently. We were more suspicious of others and more cautious. Perhaps we avoided larger events, even though we may not have been directly victimized as were those in New York, Virginia, and Washington, D.C.

Experiences do frame our thoughts (Adler, 1930). If you tell me you are a friend but you hurt me, I will not think of you as a friend. My private logic regarding you becomes, "You are not to be trusted, you are not safe because of the experience I had with you."

Traumatized children develop a complex list of thoughts, a private logic, as a result of their experiences. One example of the private logic that develops in children who have been abused is, "I will fight any person that I feel is a threat to me, any person who tries to control me because if I do not, I will be hurt again, and again and again."

Following are the completed private logic statements presented at the beginning of this chapter. How do your answers compare?

> ➤ I must do something to let you know I am terrified.
> ➤ I will do whatever I need to do in order to control you and your responses to me in order to survive.
> ➤ I will fight any experienced activity, any person that tries to control me because if I let you control me, I am vulnerable to your abuse and your abandonment again and again.
> ➤ I will not do what you want me to do because if I do and do not do well, you will ridicule me, berate me, abuse me, or abandon me.

Attempting to reassure terrified children with words alone rarely helps reverse their private logic. Private logic is created by previous experiences and will only be altered or replaced with a different, hopefully strength-based logic as a result of new experiences that sometimes need to be experienced repeatedly. This will be discussed in detail in the next chapter when we address the importance of self-regulation.

Survival Behaviors Driven by Experiences

Survival behaviors are also formed, driven, and repeated because of how children experienced past traumatic situations and how they are experiencing their current situation, environment, and people in their environment. When children feel unsafe, threatened, or powerless, trauma-related survival behaviors are likely to result. When children are direct victims of repeated trauma, like abuse, or exposed to multiple traumas, survival behaviors become more acute and include primitive, survival-directed fight, flight, and freeze behaviors (as detailed in Chapter 1). DTD criteria include these survival responses, but they also present a wider range of experiences than specified in the current PTSD diagnostic category. Problems with self-harm, self-soothing, risk-taking, trust, reciprocity, support seeking, and affect regulation are a few of the areas not addressed in the current PTSD diagnostic category (van der Kolk et al., 2009).

In essence, when children are engaged in survival behaviors, it is because they are terrified by someone or something in their environment and simply know of no other way to respond. At this moment of activation, children need to experience something that is calming, soothing, familiar, and safe—something they have engaged in previously that has allowed them to feel safe and in control and that regulates their physiological, behavioral, and emotional reactions. Talk rarely fills this need. Being with someone they feel safe with, going to a place where they feel safe, doing something they feel safe doing, and having what helps calm them is what they need to experience in order to regain control and regulate their reactions. Therefore, it becomes essential that the healing process and healing environment be trauma-informed, understand the survival needs of traumatized children, and be able to provide the resources and opportunities for children to easily access the *who* and *what* that allow them to experience a renewed sense of control and safety (Steele & Malchiodi, 2012; van der Kolk et al., 1996; van der Kolk, 2009).

The Primary Differences

Table 2.1 presented a list of the primary differences we have been discussing. In the next chapter we present the same table but add to it the body's reactions to grief and trauma within a trauma-informed context. This will help us to also further appreciate the need to teach children to resource their bodies in order to regulate their responses to extreme stress. In reality it can be difficult at times to determine whether children are experiencing grief, trauma, or both until we have spent some time with children in their world. We developed the *SITCAP* intervention process based on the ways children often experience their losses and traumas.

A Magical Moment

I am happy to share a magical moment I had with a 15-year-old male client I was seeing for an extensive trauma history, including living with a mom who was crack addicted, prostituted out of their home, the family dumpster dived to get food, and mom was physically and verbally abusive; my client had been in 11 foster homes between the ages of 8 and 15, and in one of them a boy molested him. He presented with ADHD symptoms, depression, and behavioral problems. He also had enuresis.

He was somewhat resistant to doing the drawings; frankly, he was somewhat resistant to any therapy, having been in therapy since he was placed out of his home. He had very little faith in therapy being helpful, because his oppositional and defiant behaviors were always the focus of treatment rather than how he was actually experiencing his world.

After the third session with *SITCAP*, the enuresis was extinguished—permanently. Behavioral concerns were much reduced, as reported by his then foster mother, and over the summer he was able to retain his placement and build an amicable relationship with his foster mother. *SITCAP* has been invaluable for the teen boys I have seen as well as for myself.

Sabina Alasti-Ward, MEd, PCC, SIBR Program Coordinator,
Child and Adolescent Behavioral Health, Canton, Ohio

Summary

The nature of children's experiences are at the core of their world and, therefore, should be at the core of what guides us in determining what will be most helpful. Intervention must begin with experiences that meet the needs of traumatized children in their world. Those experiences must always be safe, empowering, and directed at altering the way children view themselves, others, and the world around them. For this to happen, intervention must be trauma-informed, address the major experiences of trauma, and be structured in ways to influence changes in the thoughts and behaviors associated with trauma to those associated with being a survivor, a thriver, resilient, and ready to flourish. In the following chapter, we present the key principles of trauma-informed care and their integration into the *SITCAP* model.

Three

Trauma-Informed Principles and Practices

In the first two chapters, we cited research supporting the efficacy of *SITCAP's* (*Structured Sensory Interventions for Traumatized Children, Adolescents and Parents*) primary use of sensory-based interventions to help children with the sensations, feelings, and images created by their traumatic experiences. This chapter further discusses the need for sensory intervention, the role of the right hemisphere and implicit processing in the intervention process, the relationship between drawing and the externalization of children's iconic memories, as well as the releasing of the physiological memories stored in the body. Once the need for sensory interventions is established, it is equally important to establish *SITCAP* as a trauma-informed process. Trauma-informed practice criteria are presented, along with the ways these criteria are integrated into *SITCAP*. This chapter is the final chapter establishing our intervention as a trauma-informed practice while also establishing the rationale for the specific intervention activities to be detailed and illustrated in subsequent chapters.

Being Trauma-Informed

The development of the National Center for Trauma-Informed Care (NCTIC) in 2011 marked a new era in our understanding of the impact of trauma on children and its implications for treatment. Table 3.1 provides a list of terms and trauma treatment models that are frequently written about in trauma-focused articles and books. Being trauma-informed suggests that we ought to be able to discuss in detail the important role and value each of these terms and models plays in providing trauma-informed care and initiating trauma-informed practices. This is not an all-inclusive listing, but it does begin to reflect the scope of what we know about childhood trauma today and what is needed to guide and support the care and treatment of traumatized children.

Being trauma-informed is an ethical responsibility as our new knowledge supported by science is redirecting our understanding of what matters most to traumatized children's efforts to survive and flourish despite their traumatic histories. Neuroscience has moved us, in a relatively short period of time, from thinking that children do not experience trauma to knowing that they are vulnerable to a full range of trauma-specific

Table 3.1   Trauma Terms

▪ Safety	▪ Neuroplasticity
▪ Choice	▪ Hyperarousal
▪ Trauma-informed assessments/ relationships/environments, resilience	▪ Self-regulation
▪ Posttraumatic growth (PTG)	▪ Cortisol, oxytocin
▪ Epigenetics	▪ Iconic symbolization
▪ Exposure	▪ Sensory integration
▪ Trauma narrative	▪ Developmental Trauma Disorder (DTD)
▪ Cognitive reframing	▪ Trauma-Focused Cognitive-Behavioral Therapy (TF-CBT)
▪ Repressive coping	▪ Eye Movement Desensitization Reprocessing (EMDR)
▪ Private logic	▪ Somatic Experiencing (SE)
▪ Explicit/implicit processes	▪ Sensorimotor Psychotherapy
▪ Left and right hemispheres	▪ *Structured Sensory Intervention for Traumatized Children, Adolescents and Parents (SITCAP)*
▪ The triune brain	▪ Neurosequential Model of Therapeutics (NMT)
▪ Thinking/feeling/survival brain	▪ Trauma Incident Reduction (TIR)
▪ Amygdala	▪ Mindfulness, trauma integration
▪ Hippocampus	
▪ Frontal cortex	
▪ Broca's area	

reactions. The Chowchilla School Bus kidnapping in California made national headlines in 1976. When the 26 children who were buried alive in their school bus were rescued, doctors examined the children, found them in good health, and sent them home. They did not request mental health intervention (Terr, 1994). Even when children were included in the *DSM-IV* PTSD category in 1994, there was minimal acceptance that children could experience the range of PTSD reactions we once only attributed to adult survivors of war. Today we know that children do experience the full range of reactions listed under PTSD in the *DSM-IV-TR* (APA, 2000), and also the even more expansive list of reactions presented in the proposed DTD cited earlier.

The Need for Sensory-Based Interventions

Technological advances allowing the *lens* of neuroscience to see how the brain and the body experience extreme stress, fear, and terror have also led to accepting that sensory-based interventions do help traumatized children. They specifically help with the non-cognitive aspects of their traumatic experiences, which when not attended to do contribute to the many reactions assigned to trauma (Foa, Keene, Friedman, & Cohen, 2008).

SITCAP's sensory-based healing approach helps externalize the *iconic images* stored implicitly and assists the body in finding relief from the stored biological and physiological reactions of that trauma experience, neither of which responds well to cognitive approaches alone. We begin with Witness Justice (2010), a resource for victims, which summarizes the impact of trauma in their health and wellness section under the title, *Trauma Is the Common Denominator: New Discoveries in the Science of Traumatic Behavior*:

> When experienced in childhood, trauma produces neurobiological impacts on the brain causing dysfunction in the hippocampus, amygdala, medial frontal cortex and other limbic structures. When confronted with danger, the brain moves from a normal information-processing state to a survival-oriented, reactive alarm state. Trauma causes the body's nervous system to experience: an extreme adrenaline rush; intense fear; information processing problems; and a severe reduction or shutdown of cognitive capacities.

Discussions related to the cognitive limitations of traumatized children have taken place for many years. Lenore Terr, the author of *Too Scared to Cry* (1990), reported that memories of traumatized individuals are far more emotional and perceptual in content than declarative components. In *Traumatic Stress*, van der Kolk, McFarlane, and Weisaeth (1996) observed that when a terrifying incident such as trauma is experienced and does not fit into a contextual memory, a new memory or dissociation is established, and memories are "stored initially as sensory fragments that have no linguistic components" (p. 289). This collection of terror-based, nonlinguistic components drives that child's behavior. The *shutting down* of cognitive capacities dictates the use of a nonlanguage, sensory-based approach such as *SITCAP* to help the traumatized child with what he has no words to describe and that reason and logic cannot explain or change. *SITCAP*'s sensory approach, as detailed in earlier chapters, helps to override and/or replace the trauma-associated sensory fragments with the kind of sensory memories that can induce strength-based, resilience-focused contextual memories.

Storing the Implicit Memories of Trauma

The developmental, cognitive, and verbal challenges of children support that cognitive-behavioral approaches may be limited in their efforts to help traumatized children. Gil (2006) notes that traumatic events are experienced and stored *implicitly* in the right hemisphere of the brain (where there is no language, reason, logic) and that "this suggests that allowing children a period of time to access and stimulate the right hemisphere of the brain could eventually activate the necessary (explicit) functions of the left hemisphere, which appears to shut down during traumatic experiences" (p. 102). When people are in extreme fear, the right brain shuts down the capacity of our thinking brain. Perry (2004) reported that traumatized students often hear only about half the words spoken by their teachers. Most of us have had the experience of being at a social event or business meeting that makes us uncomfortable. Our anxiety level is activated more than usual and, at some point, we have the experience of not being able to recall the name of someone we know or an important business fact pertinent to our meeting. The harder we try to engage our cognitive (left) brain, the more difficult it becomes to remember and the more our anxiety increases. Later, when in a safer environment, doing what we feel comfortable doing, we suddenly remember.

SITCAP implicitly engages the right brain, using safe and calming activities that later allow for left-brain engagement to support the cognitive reframing of one's experiences. In Chapter 1, for example, Tables 1.1 through 1.6 indicated significant reductions in disso-ciation and thought problems in cases involving chronic abuse and witness to domestic violence. In severe cases involving early delayed development of cognitive processes, intervention will need to be directed at developmentally appropriate remedial intervention regarding cognitive processes. Although we do not discuss what constitutes a compre-hensive, trauma-informed assessment in this work, in severe cases a neurodevelopment evaluation is critical to applying interventions that address delayed neurodevelopment,

---

Point of Interest

All About the Brain

As trauma specialists, we have to understand how trauma impacts the brain to effectively work with traumatized youth. When it comes to the brain and trauma, there are countless facts and concepts to remember.

Some important brain facts to remember include the following:

➢ A fetus is impacted by an increase in maternal stress. Maternal cortisol levels pass through the placenta and raise the heart rate and cortisol levels in the unborn fetus.

➢ Because of an intense surge in stress hormones, the brains of traumatized children are not as well integrated as the brains of nontraumatized children. This helps explain why traumatized children have significant difficulties with learning, emotional regulation, integrated functioning, and social development.

➢ It takes at least 5 minutes for a new neuronal (brain) connection to form, hence the importance of repetition when providing interventions.

➢ The brain isn't fully developed until the end of adolescence—age 23!

➢ Each experience, whether good or bad, creates new neuronal connections in our brain. Experience becomes our biology.

➢ Our brains are constantly changing. This is why it is never too late to provide a child with repetitive, new, positive experiences.

such as sensory integration, language, speech, and social cognitive skills. For a detailed discussion as to what constitutes a trauma-informed assessment, we recommend *Trauma-Informed Practices with Children and Adolescents* (Steele & Malchiodi, 2012).

Because the right brain is tied to the amygdala, it is more fear based. The amygdala is like a smoke detector: When it senses danger, it sets off an alarm. It reads and responds to facial expressions and tone of voice, not language (Brendtro, Mitchell, McCall, 2009). We may be very skilled practitioners, but if we have physical features similar to the person who did that bad thing to a child, the child's alarm will be set off, and he will not feel safe with us. Traumatized children live in the right hemisphere, the limbic region where life is experienced *implicitly* at a sensory level, not *explicitly* at a cognitive level. This is why it becomes important to help the child with sensory experiences that calm his fears. Ogden, Minton, and Pain (2006) write:

> In a psychotherapeutic setting, focusing primarily on word-based thinking and narratives can keep therapy at a surface level and trauma may be unresolved. . . . Within an interpersonal neurobiology view of therapy, as we "sift" the mind, we attempt to integrate the sensations, images, feelings and thoughts that compromise the flow of energy and information that defines our mental lives. (p. xiv)

Iconic Images of Trauma

Focusing on the internalized, iconic images, which reflect the way children relate to their world, is an approach that dates back at least to Carl Jung. Jung split from Freud in 1912 in part because of their difference of opinion about fantasies: "Jung believed that if one took the images and symbols of the unconscious as valid and related to them as such, then the inner life would unfold and develop" (Allan, 1988, p. 3). Using drawing as a way for children to present their iconic memories, Pynoos and Eth (1986) initiated a brief, one-session drawing activity to help children who had been exposed to violence to more easily communicate how they experienced that violence. *SITCAP* has demonstrated repeatedly that when we see what traumatized children see when they look at themselves and life, we discover what matters most to their efforts to heal. In Chapter 2 we talked about the iconic images that shape the traumatized child's view of self and drive behavior. When children perceive their world to be threatening, they engage in the kind of survival behaviors detailed in the previous chapter. Real or not, these images/fantasies do bring their inner world to life in the form of behavior.

Because these iconic images are implicitly stored in the right brain, it becomes essential that we help children develop stronger images of themselves as survivors and of others and life as nonthreatening. Again, this is not possible using word-based cognitive approaches. Steele (2003) notes that:

When memory cannot be linked linguistically in a contextual framework, it remains at a symbolic (iconic) level where there are no words to describe it, only sensations and images. Before traumatic memory can be encoded, expressed through language, and successfully integrated, it must be retrieved and implicitly externalized in its symbolic (iconic) sensory forms. (p. 142)

Malchiodi (2008) supports that trauma experiences are "more easily communicated through imagery and activities associated with the sensory experiences of those incidents than through cognitive processes" (p. 3).

Externalizing Implicit Memories by Drawing

SITCAP uses drawing as the primary vehicle for externalizing, revealing, and altering as needed the iconic images shaped by children's traumatic experiences. Drawing is not a new medium for children to reveal their inner world. Riley (1997) indicated that the act of drawing served as a form of externalization, a way for children to put the experience outside of themselves, to make it real and concrete. Drawing becomes a way for us, the practitioners, to see what children see as they look at themselves and the world around them. Beyers (1996) noted that numerous studies have illustrated that the use of drawings helped children access, reveal, and heal from their traumatic memories. Magwaza, Killian, Peterson, and Pillay (1993) achieved similar results with South African children who had been exposed to community violence. Saigh and Bremner (1999) suggested "that children draw sketches of their stressful experience and verbally repeat the content of their experiences" (p. 370).

Following 9/11, the World Trade Center Children's Mural Project was unveiled on March 19, 2002, and depicted more than 3,100 portraits that "served to lessen feelings of isolation and helplessness felt among those children who had difficulty understanding cognitively the complexity of this tragedy" (Berberian, Bryant, & Landsberg, 2003). Gil (2003) indicated that what might be experienced in the brain as disorganized or chaotic may, through drawing, then take on qualities of something that is manageable. What makes drawing unique in the *SITCAP* programs is its use to depict the varied ways in which children experienced what happened and/or how they are experiencing life since the trauma, if addressing the trauma is too difficult or there is no specific memory of what happened. It is also used to create new images of self and life that are strength-based and resilience-focused in order to help children better self-regulate their responses to everyday life. Chapter 4 describes the therapeutic benefits of drawing within the structured process of the *SITCAP* program.

The Body in Trauma

Bessel van der Kolk (1994) wrote an article for the *Harvard Review of Psychiatry* titled "The Body Keeps the Score: Memory and the Evolving Psychobiology of Posttraumatic

Stress." He noted that the body retains a memory of that traumatic event as much as the brain does, and that memory forms in response to the body's efforts to escape that trauma. He goes on to recommend that "For therapy to be effective it might be useful to focus on the patient's physical self-experience and increase their self-awareness, rather than focusing exclusively on the meaning that people make of their experience" (p. 13). Ogden et al. (2006) posit that this body memory largely results from the experience of trauma being stored as procedural memory. Procedural memory is a type of implicit or sensory-based memory, and it is the most basic and primitive form of memory. As the name implies, this is the type of memory for procedures or for basic associations between stimuli and responses. For example, the process or procedure for riding a bike is stored as procedural memory. Once the procedure is learned, by making the association between stimulus and appropriate responses, it is stored as a procedural memory.

Trauma-specific memories are also procedural memories and involve unconscious sensorimotor responses (Scaer, 2005) based on an individual's past experiences. Therefore, the past experience unconsciously drives the way a person with PTSD responds to current experiences. Procedural memory often leaves trauma survivors with a somatic or body experience that is linked to overwhelming body sensations, negative emotion, and maladaptive thoughts that are all easily activated by internal and external triggers (Langmuir, Kirsh, & Classen, 2012). These triggers often negatively impact a traumatized individual's ability to regulate emotions and control behavior. For example, an adolescent with a history of physical abuse may respond to a supportive touch on the shoulder as a threat. Before even realizing what he is doing, the touch elicits a body memory that triggers him to respond with a fight response in the form of aggressive hitting of the person who is only trying to offer a gesture of encouragement. Therefore, this is processed as an emotional experience, without thought or logic, but rather driven by a body response to the past trauma memory.

In *Trauma-Informed Practices with Children and Adolescents* (Steele & Malchiodi, 2012), Peter Levine explained this differently when he wrote:

> trauma is a physiological phenomenon, rather than a purely psychological one. As such, psychologists, psychiatrists, and other helping professionals need to understand the core mechanisms of how to stabilize the body's reactions to traumatic stress on the physical level in order to help children and teens regulate their sensations and emotions. (p. 5)

Levine also wrote:

> When children's physiological survival systems are activated by threat, the excess energy used to defend oneself must be expended. If that energy is not fully

discharged and metabolized, it does not simply disappear. Instead it remains as a kind of highly charged body memory creating the potential for repeated traumatic symptoms. (p. 4)

Today there is consensus that trauma is a mind/body experience that necessitates a mind/body approach to help regulate the reactions to trauma experiences past and present (Siegel, 2007). Emotional regulation is the development of the ability to maintain a well-regulated emotional state in coping with everyday stress. Increasing awareness of experiences, emotions, and body sensations may be helpful to traumatized youth, because the practice can enhance emotion regulation and limit reactivity (Gratz & Roemer, 2004; Heller & Lapierre, 2012; Linehan et al., 2010). The ability to differentiate between emotions and body sensations has been related to effective emotion regulation. If a person can discriminate between his or her emotions, he or she would be more likely to notice specific body sensations that are connected to emotions (Hill & Updegraff, 2012). Table 3.2 presents Levine and Kline's additions to the original comparisons made by TLC and illustrated in Chapter 2. The asterisk indicates the additions they made in

Table 3.2   The Inclusion of the Nervous System's Reactions to Trauma

Grief	Trauma
Generalized reaction: SADNESS	Generalized reaction: TERROR
Grief reactions can stand alone.	Trauma reactions generally also include grief reactions.
Grief reactions are generally known to the public and the professional.	Trauma reactions, especially in children, are largely unknown to the public and often to professionals.
In grief, guilt says, "I wish I would or would not have . . . "	Trauma guilt says, "It was my fault. I could have prevented it. It should have been me."
Grief generally does not attack or "disfigure" our identity.	Trauma generally attacks, distorts, and "disfigures" our identity. *our self-image and confidence
In grief, dreams tend to be of the person who died.	In trauma, dreams are about the child him or her self dying or being hurt. *with nightmarish images
In grief, pain is related to the loss.	In trauma, pain is related to the tremendous terror and an overwhelming sense of powerlessness and fear for safety.
In grief, a child's anger is generally not destructive. *nonviolent	In trauma, a child's anger often becomes assaultive (even after nonviolent trauma, fighting often increases). * anger often becomes violent to others or self (substance use, spousal and child abuse)
*In grief, talking can be a relief.	*In trauma, talking is difficult or impossible.
*Grief is healed through emotional release.	*Trauma is healed through the nervous system.
*Grief reactions diminish over time.	*Trauma symptoms may worsen over time and develop into PTSD and/or health problems.

Trauma reactions are DIFFERENT from grief reactions
Trauma reactions OVERPOWER grief reactions

Children can be traumatized by violent or nonviolent incidents. Separation from a parent through divorce or foster care, a family member's terminal illness or sudden death, exposure to physical or sexual abuse, witness of drug use, surviving a house fire, experiencing extreme weather such as tornados, floods, earthquakes, or hurricanes, as well as witnessing drowning, murder, suicide, and school violence can all be traumatizing incidents.

*Differences added by Levine and Kline (2007).

their publication, *Trauma Through a Child's Eyes* (Levine & Kline, 2007). These additions reflect the nervous system's reaction to trauma, which often needs regulating.

Actively Involving Children in Their Own Healing

The *SITCAP* process involves children in their own healing process. It helps them to define where in their bodies they are experiencing what happened to them, what that is like (in concrete terms), who or what makes it worse, and who or what makes it better. The entire process allows children to discover how to create safe places using their body as a resource. It teaches them that, even though there may be constant reminders in their environment of that bad thing that happened or is still happening, they can regulate their body's response and subsequently their feelings in ways that support their capacity to manage the challenges they face. Several intervention strategies address each of these sensory issues. *SITCAP* is designed as a short-term, integrated approach for addressing the iconic images, sensations, feelings, and cognitive changes induced by trauma. It is directed at overriding the trauma-driven sensory memories and sensations with strength-based, resilience-focused sensory experiences and memories that become the more dominant response to life's daily challenges. However, to support the primary dictate of trauma-informed care, "Do no harm" (Hodas, 2006), the intervention process must be guided by the core principles of trauma-informed care.

Trauma-Informed Principles and Practices

The core principles of trauma-informed care recorded by the NCTIC (2011) address the responsibility of childcare delivery systems and organizations. They include:

Understanding trauma and its impact
Promoting safety
Ensuring cultural competence
Supporting consumer control, choice, and autonomy
Healing happens in relationships
Integrating care
Understanding recovery is possible

Promoting trauma-informed care at the system level continues to bring about major changes in delivery systems that are now more sensitive to the needs of traumatized children, thanks to the effort of the NCTIC and its many divisions. *Practice* refers to the specific methods we use to help traumatized children in our care, how we approach the intervention process, relate to the child, and provide the intervention. The intervention itself should meet the criteria presented in Chapter 1 as to what supports an evidence-based intervention. The seven core criteria of trauma-informed practice presented here are those criteria most frequently addressed in the plethora of articles on best practices and research regarding trauma and trauma-informed care:

1. Restore a sense of safety, empowerment, and self-regulation.
2. Integrate implicit and explicit processes.
3. Apply neurodevelopmentally appropriate interventions.
4. Include interventions that respect and support cultural diversity.
5. Recognize that no one intervention fits every situation and respond appropriately.
6. Promote trauma-informed relationships and environments.
7. Promote posttraumatic growth and resilience.

Each of these seven criteria is integrated into the *SITCAP* intervention process and practice. They provide for a structured approach that is directed at keeping the intervention safe for children but also for the practitioner. How *SITCAP* meets the criteria that support the intervention as a trauma-informed practice demands additional discussion.

Safety, Empowerment, and Self-Regulation

Bath (2008) refers to safety, empowerment, and self-regulation as the three pillars of trauma-informed care. If one pillar is missing in our effort to help, it weakens the overall healing effort. In many ways they are interconnected. When we help children feel a greater sense of safety, they will feel more empowered, but they also experience longer periods of calm, thereby strengthening their self-regulation capacity. When children learn that they can regulate their reactions, they feel both empowered and safe. *SITCAP* uses several processes directed at strengthening each of these pillars.

Safety

➢ By beginning and ending each session in a safe place, we are teaching children to regulate their responses. By containing the trauma focus within these *safety bookends*, we are also regulating the overall experience for children into more easily manageable segments. This consistent and predictable process allows children to feel safer.

➢ The trauma-specific questions used in *SITCAP* to explore how children are experiencing their lives are open-ended. They keep the practitioner in the role of being curious but also allow children to guide the process and, in so doing, to feel safer. When children are asked closed-ended questions, they often become suspicious, which in turn triggers more of a survival response, in this case shutting down. Olfason and Kenniston's (2008) research reveals that "open-ended questions are the most productive even reluctant or non-disclosing children respond to the most" (p. 77).

➢ The nonlanguage, sensory-based activities of *SITCAP* afford children an additional sense of safety, because they can express themselves without using language. For some children, any form of questioning may be difficult to respond to and increase anxiety.

➤ Practitioners do not take notes during the sessions, because to do so makes it difficult for the practitioner to remain actively curious. Note taking also potentially increases children's anxiety and fear that they may reveal too much, not say the "right thing," or that the practitioner is going to tell others about what was said. This significantly reduces children's sense of safety.

➤ All too often we are in a hurry to interpret and reflect our wisdom to children rather than allowing children in their time to arrive at what matters most to them. The structure of *SITCAP* supports following the lead of children—not interpreting, but instead listening and acknowledging—while we stay in their world, moving at their pace. Empowering children in this way brings them a greater sense of safety.

➤ *SITCAP*'s sensory activities are contained within an 8-by-11 sheet of paper. Fine point pencils and markers are used to provide greater detail while restricting psychomotor activity. What we mean by this is that the activities do not involve larger psychomotor activity or expressive mediums that tend to trigger more expressive reactions, which increase the risk for emotional flooding. "A little at a time" is the consistent theme of the *SITCAP* process. In addition, each session begins and ends in the same way, so the process becomes predictable. Predictability for traumatized children is essential for and equivalent to safety.

Empowerment

➤ When children do not feel safe with the intervention process, they resist responding. Because we believe children are the best experts about what is helping or hurting them, we empower them to lead the intervention process. We made several references to the child's ability to say *yes* or *no* to any part of our effort to help. We all agree that having a choice is empowering. When focusing on the trauma, children are also free or empowered to tell whatever they would like to tell or select whatever incident they wish.

➤ Children are empowered by being given multiple opportunities to express what matters most to them without relying on words to do so. The range of sensory-based activities in *SITCAP* provides these opportunities.

➤ In the *SITCAP* process, children are also given multiple opportunities to bring us into their world, to take us where they decide to take us. Giving children this opportunity to be our teacher and our guide, they become empowered. The more they experience a sense of empowerment, the safer they feel and the more they can begin to regulate their reactions to extreme stress.

➤ Empowerment is directly related to what we believe about ourself, others, and our life. Children of trauma experience life as victims, others as constant threats, and life as terrifying. The entire *SITCAP* process is about engaging children in experiences that alter the subjective view of self as victims to that as survivors and thrivers. When children experience this change, they are naturally empowered to redefine themselves and their lives from a strength/resilience perspective, as seen in the sample cases we present.

There is no doubt that for some severely traumatized children this is only a beginning; they will need repeated support beyond the *SITCAP* program. However, even in our study of those children who did not do as well as other traumatized children participating in *SITCAP*, even the smallest iconic shift from seeing self as a victim to that of a potential survivor resulted in significant gains as reported by children and their parents, teachers, and social workers (Steele et al., 2009).

Self-Regulation

Self-regulation refers to mastery over one's unwanted reactions to extreme stress. *SITCAP* supports varied and repeated processes that teach and reinforce self-regulation.

➤ Choice; the use of resources and mediums like music, play, and so on; and activities that use the body as a resource all assist with the development of self-regulation mastery. Within the *SITCAP* process, children are encouraged to stop doing what may be inducing too much anxiety and immediately go to the resource or activity that is calming or deactivating. Children learn that when they change what they are doing, seeing, or thinking about themselves, they can feel better. The ability to practice these strategies teaches children that they can regulate overwhelming and uncomfortable reactions.

➤ Beginning and ending each session in a safe place also reinforces self-regulation behaviors by titrating the trauma focus within a safe, structured, and predictable framework.

➤ Safety, predictability, and consistency have always been essential to the development of emotional stability or self-regulation (Perry, 2012). These are the elements framing the *SITCAP* process.

Practitioners are taught to help children become attuned to how their bodies are reacting to what they are doing, feeling, and thinking about. *SITCAP*'s trauma-informed questions help practitioners help children become more attuned to their bodies. One example of how these questions help resource the body is related to our focus on *hurt*. The following questions help children attend to their internal reactions, as well as their ability to regulate and change reactions when needed. Some of the questions included in *SITCAP* are:

➤ Where do you feel the hurt the most in your body?
➤ What does it make you want to do?
➤ What do you do that helps make the hurt go away?
➤ How big or small is your hurt?
➤ How big or small is that hurt now (after intervention)?

Using this process, children are reminded to continue using what they have found that makes the hurt better, as long as it is not self-defeating. The practitioner also learns through this process what other activities children may need so they have multiple ways to self-regulate.

Although *SITCAP* is itself a self-regulatory process, some children may need a longer-term use of a variety of methods beyond *SITCAP* to strengthen their self-regulation efforts, especially when children remain in environments that are traumatic. Self-regulation can be supported by many nontherapeutic activities. Lakes and Hoyt (2004) conducted a study in which elementary-aged children were evaluated before and after taking Tae Kwon Do training over a 3-month period. Compared to the control group, these children had greater improvement in cognitive affect and physical control, better classroom conduct, better socialization, and improvement on a math test.

Music has repeatedly proven to be an excellent way to strengthen self-regulation (Davis, 2010; Gao, 2008). Mindfulness has also proven helpful in efforts to self-regulate (Cahn & Polich, 2006). Involving children in activities where they need to use their hands to create something can also be calming and soothing (Malchiodi, 2008). Somatic Experiencing (Levine & Kline, 2008) and Sensorimotor Psychotherapy (Ogden et al., 2006) are also excellent processes that focus on self-regulation by using the body as a resource.

Integrating Implicit and Explicit Processes

We begin *SITCAP* by meeting traumatized children where they are living and processing their world—predominantly in the right hemisphere, midbrain region, sometimes referred to as the *survival brain*, where there is no reason or logic. Our effort is to externalize these subjective experiences and transform them into a concrete form that then allows children the opportunity to cognitively reorder them in ways they can now manage. In essence, we want to bring about an integrated balance between the use of right and left hemispheres, between the thinking brain and the survival brain. This balance allows us to successfully manage our environments and our lives.

Recent studies in neuroscience indicate that both the left and right hemispheres are involved in almost all cognitive tasks and that emotions play a critical role in what is learned (Chen, Moran, & Gardner, 2009). This said, neuroscience also shows that "learning anything requires building new neural networks [by] being actively involved in what is being learned" (Fischer, 2012). The *SITCAP* process directs itself at actively involving children in new experiences in order for them to build new neural networks related to what they are learning about themselves and trauma as a result of the sensory-based activities they engage in when participating in *SITCAP*. These activities bring about new strength-based and resilience-focused emotional outcomes that further help them understand and integrate what is being learned. The processes we have used over the past 23 years are now being supported by what neuroscience is confirming about how we learn (not memorize) and how we actually integrate our experiences between right and left hemispheres in ways that give our subjective experiences personal meaning, function, and purpose.

➤ What makes *SITCAP* unique is that structured sensory-based activities lead to positive strength-based and resilience-focused cognitive conclusions by the children who engage in these activities. *SITCAP* activities become the silent right hemisphere (brain) teacher that presents thoughts that are difficult to reject because those thoughts about self, others, and the world naturally emerge from the activities the children experience. These thoughts are then reinforced with cognitive reframing statements specific to what was experienced in that session and are therefore more acceptable to children.

➤ Right and left hemispheres are involved consistently in every session. The *Who I AM* activity, for example, is a sensory activity that allows children to validate that many parts make them who they are, that trauma is only one part of their life, and that trauma does not define them. Many of their "parts" will be strengths that can be consistently reinforced. Reframing what they have learned through completing the activity further elaborates and confirms that they can use these resources to help them face very difficult times and help them thrive despite their trauma.

➤ This process is repeated in every session as a way to repetitively influence children to remember that their thoughts (private logic), feelings, and behaviors are governed by their experiences and their view of self, others, and the world. To change the unwanted feelings, thoughts, and related behaviors, they learn that they need to change the experience.

Appropriate Developmental Intervention

Infants and children need to experience attunement through comforting and reassuring touch; repeated eye contact; kind, pleasant, and soothing words; predictability; and physical and emotional safety for optimal development. When these needs are not met as a result of traumatic experiences, children experience developmental trauma (van der Kolk, 2005). Developmental trauma is often manifested by hyperactivity and out-of-control, troubling behaviors that repeatedly challenge the patience of children's parents, practitioners, and systems such as schools. Depending on the frequency of experiences, developmental trauma behaviors such as bullying, chronic lying, self-mutilation, and disturbed attachment can become far more risky (Weinhold & Weinhold, 2009). Testing limits is the way children let us know they do not feel safe. Setting limits and engaging in sensory activities that are attuned to the developmental needs of traumatized children is necessary. We again encourage readers to study the proposed DTD to appreciate the complexities associated with developmental trauma (van der Kolk et al., 2009). Many of the children who have participated in *SITCAP* met the DTD criteria. Although many of these children needed additional intervention, *SITCAP* helped them experience significant gains, making it far easier for them to continue with additional intervention, especially within the structured use of other expressive interventions. Following are the ways *SITCAP* approaches developmental areas:

> *SITCAP* programs are written and designed to appropriately match the developmental ranges of children 6 to 18 years old.

> Practitioners are trained to direct their interventions toward children's developmental level, not chronological age. Some children who are 13 or 14 and who are developmentally delayed may do better with activities designed for younger children.

Magical Moment

SITCAP is a treatment modality that allows for our troubled youth at Pressley Ridge to safely work through their relational trauma. One of our teens, age 15, has a history of trauma filled with abuse, neglect, substance abuse, and domestic violence. Prior to her trauma intervention, she often verbalized frequent self-deprecating thoughts and struggled to see the hope in overcoming the traumas that have haunted her for years. Toward the end of her treatment work, there was an incident the night before a *SITCAP* session where she experienced a trauma reaction at family dinner night with her older brother, who was also a Pressley Ridge resident and experienced much of the same abuse that his sister had experienced. The trauma reaction was triggered when a male resident was staring at her. When looking for emotional support from her brother, her brother lost his cool and started making threats to hurt this male resident, which only intensified her anxiety and distress. When processing this trauma reaction the next day, it was discussed and determined that she and her brother would benefit from a family session.

The family session was empowering and strengthening for both the brother and sister. The session accomplished two exciting things: (1) it provided a vehicle for the sister to teach her brother how to recognize and respond to her when she is activated; and (2) most importantly, her brother, who also struggles with his own trauma, was able to witness and experience the strength of his sister in overcoming the hold the trauma has had on her throughout her life as a result of participating in *SITCAP*. Subsequently, it served to motivate her brother to work on his own treatment of past trauma. The *SITCAP* program effectively allows our kids to face their trauma and create a release for the trauma memories that are locked in their bodies. Michelle and several other residents have shown a strong reduction in symptoms and an overall improvement in self-concept and confidence.

Douglas Pfeifer, MA, LPC, ALPS; Clinical Coordinator, Pressley Ridge at White Oak, West Virginia; and Alison Finch, MS, Provisionally Licensed Counselor, Clinical Supervisor/Therapist at Pressley Ridge

Although assessment is not discussed in any detail in this book, if a 13-year-old is assessed to be functioning cognitively at a first-grade level, then the activities for that developmental level are selected.

➤ Taking a history of developmental markers, along with trauma incident timelines, can alert us to possible developmental and neurological delays and the need for more extensive evaluation. Certainly one of the values of focusing on children's experiences is that we discover explanations for their behaviors that, in a trauma-informed context, make perfect sense while providing us information to select the developmentally appropriate activities.

We must remain alert to the fact that early trauma can induce several cognitive and sensory integration delays that impede healing if they are not addressed along with trauma. History taking and initial trauma-related screening is conducted in the initial *SITCAP* session with children and, when possible, separately with their parents/ guardians. The need for a more extensive evaluation is based on indicators that emerge during the program that suggest the need for further evaluation. Ideally, a complete trauma-informed assessment is preferred, but may not be possible in many cases for several practical reasons. We acknowledge that severe developmental trauma will need intervention beyond the use of *SITCAP*. When additional intervention is needed, practitioners are reminded to present those interventions within the kind of structured framework used with *SITCAP*. The continued use of expressive interventions with cognitive-based interventions, within this structured framework of *SITCAP*, is also encouraged.

Supporting Cultural Diversity

SITCAP engages in several processes that support its sensitivity to the critical influences of diversity on the healing process:

➤ *SITCAP* requires practitioners to explain in detail the intervention process and to empower children to feel comfortable saying *yes* or *no* to what they are asked to do or talk about. In this way, even if the practitioner inadvertently asks children to do or talk about what is *taboo* in their culture or not a part of their worldview, children can more easily teach the practitioner what is or is not acceptable or pertinent given the customs, values, and worldview of their culture.

➤ Practitioners attempting to help children of ethnically diverse cultures have an ethical responsibility to be well-informed about that diversity. However, research (NCTSN, 2005; Snowden, Hu, & Jerrell, 1995) clearly documents that outcomes are not necessarily going to improve simply because of a practitioner's knowledge of that culture's values and customs. It does show that the best outcomes are achieved when practitioners are equally matched to the diverse group they are seeing. This makes sense, and for this reason *SITCAP* is designed so its materials can be easily translated to match the language of children without altering the process. The focus on strengths and resilience presented, for example, in the cognitive reframing component of each session may not support what other cultures define to be strengths or factors of resilience. Without altering the process, the ethnically matched practitioner can easily initiate the reframing process, referring to those strengths accepted as a value in that child's culture.

➤ *SITCAP* sessions focus on the subjective experiences universally felt by children who have been exposed to trauma-inducing situations. Fear, for example, is fear regardless of the color of our skin or our ethnicity. All children have a universal need to feel safe and empowered, and to think of themselves as being of value to others. *SITCAP* therefore naturally bridges many diverse cultures by focusing on the subjective experiences that are universal in nature.

➤ *SITCAP* relies on the medium of drawing (detailed in Chapter 4) as its primary sensory intervention process. It does provide practitioners with the option to use other sensory mediums if drawing is not something children wish to do at the time. In the drawing process, children are presented with images that are associated with the particular activity or theme being addressed in that session. These can be easily interchanged with images that are acceptable in that child's culture. In some countries, for example, the cat is seen as evil. An elephant, if acceptable, could be used in that case to help children complete that particular activity. The process does not change; the structure does not change.

The World Health Organization's *International Classification of Diseases (ICD-10)* (2012) has a diagnostic classification of trauma that represents a worldview much broader than that of the *DSM-IV-TR* classification. Because *SITCAP* does not focus on symptoms and behaviors but the ways in which children are experiencing themselves, their environment, and life as a result of trauma, it remains a valuable process regardless of international symptom assignment and cultural differences.

There Is No One Intervention

SITCAP is one intervention among many excellent interventions. It was designed to address the needs of varied populations and levels of trauma severity. However, because no one intervention fits every child, it is critical that practitioners provide children with different options when needed.

➤ The first hour of training in the use of *SITCAP* addresses the fact that interventions must *fit* the child and discusses how *SITCAP* can be integrated with other practices.

➤ As indicated earlier, we believe there is no such thing as resistance in trauma—either children feel safe or they do not. This belief also positions the practitioner to be attuned to the importance of acknowledging that some aspect of the practitioner or the environment may activate children's traumatic memories and associated fears, which may then indicate they may do better seeing someone else. This belief supports engaging a different intervention approach deemed to be more appropriate for them and also supports the importance of empowering children to say *yes* or *no*.

➤ We encourage practitioners to be cross-trained in a variety of techniques and/or to be connected to others who provide different approaches that are better suited for that child who does not feel safe, so the child has access to options. We simply consider this an ethical responsibility.

SITCAP practitioners also have access to a variety of trauma-specific resources through TLC that afford children help other than the formal *SITCAP* intervention if needed. For example, following 9/11, TLC donated thousands of copies of its grief- and trauma-focused children's book *Brave Bart: A Story for Traumatized and Grieving Children* (Sheppard, 1998). The following response from one grandmother who read the book to her granddaughter is paraphrased but reflects the kinds of responses we receive about this and other resources TLC uses to support its interventions.

I was reading *Brave Bart* to my 6-year-old granddaughter. She has been waking up frequently at night. She can be a little active but sat quietly next to me as I read the entire *Brave Bart* story. When I finished I told her she was brave just like Brave Bart said when he ended the story. She then asked me to read it again which surprised me. After a few pages my granddaughter cuddled in my lap and fell asleep before I finished the story. I took her to her bed where she slept through the night for the first time since her father, a police officer, was shot and killed a few months earlier. Thank you so much for sending *Brave Bart* to me.

Before ending this chapter, we have a brief discussion related to there being no one intervention that fits every situation. This is a wonderful example and the reason we have developed resource materials in addition to the formal *SITCAP* intervention programs. It also reflects how one person, at one brief moment in time, can have a significant impact on a child's life. Relationships are obviously critical to the success of any intervention with traumatized children. When that relationship is also a trauma-informed one, intervention progresses more easily.

Trauma-Informed Relationships

A great deal has been written about the importance of secure attachments and being connected to a significant adult as one of the strongest predictors of the child's ability to successfully bounce back from trauma and to cope with and remain at a lower risk for long-term trauma (Bowlby & Winton, 1998; Brendtro et al., 2009; Bronfenbrenner, 2005; Osofsky, 2004; Perry, 2009; Siegel, 2003).

➤ In the *SITCAP* process, the practitioner becomes the significant adult, with the intent that, in the later sessions, the practitioner brings children and their parents together so they can appreciate how their children are experiencing what has happened with them or to them, but also to help the parents respond more appropriately to their children and in so doing strengthen the connection between them.

➤ Gharabaghi (2008) says, "Relationships are the interventions" (p. 31). The qualitative study referenced earlier (Steele et al., 2009) found key differences in parent–child relationships between those who did well versus less well, although they were exposed to the same or similar traumatic experiences. When asked, "What is your favorite thing to do at home?" the children who replied "Play with my mom" did better than those who replied "Sleep" (Steele et al., 2009). *SITCAP* is about interacting with the child in his or her world. When a parent discovers how his or her child is actually experiencing the world as a result of what happened, it becomes easier to be with the child in ways that both can feel more connected. However, practitioners must also be aware that many parents of traumatized children have their own histories that are being activated by their child's trauma and that the parent may need help as well. The parent component is presented later in the text for this reason.

➤ Because *SITCAP* is structured to keep practitioners curious rather than analytical, they cannot help but be with children in their world, seeing what they see when they look at themselves, others, and the world. This level of curiosity allows children to no longer feel alone with their experiences and to be connected with an adult who is interacting and connecting implicitly with them in their world.

➤ Being curious; allowing children to bring us into their world, where and when they feel safe to do so; putting them in the role of our teachers and our guides; acknowledging rather than interpreting; providing multiple opportunities for self-expression without words; allowing them, through sensory activities, to have different implicit experiences that alter their view of self, others, and life; and, only after this, reframing what their sensory experiences taught them, contains all the practices that support efforts to develop trauma-informed relationships (Steele & Malchiodi, 2012).

Creating a Trauma-Informed Environment

The science of epigenetics has discovered that experiences within one's environment change the genetic expressions within families and across generations (Cloud, 2010; Sweatt, 2009). When an environment is experienced as safe and empowering, and where every member is treated as having value and attachments are secure, children flourish. The issues associated with creating trauma-informed environments outside of the intervention environment would consume another book. Values, beliefs, complicated system issues including family systems, affordable and accessible opportunities for strength-based experiences, and building quality connections all demand considerable attention.

> Our focus is on how the *SITCAP* process creates a trauma-informed intervention environment. It begins by honoring and practicing the pillars of trauma-informed care—safety, empowerment, and self-regulation—as detailed in the previous pages.

> We believe that children are the best experts as to what is safe for them, and giving them the opportunity to make choices is empowering.

The following list illustrates how curious queries and choices can be used to involve children in helping to make the intervention environment safe:

> When you look around the room, what in this room or about this room do you like the best?

> In this room, you can sit wherever and however you would like. Tell me, where would you like me to sit?

> Are there things you would like to bring with you the next time we meet that you really like and enjoy?

> What do you do when you get really upset?

> What do you do to feel better?

> What helps you feel better? What in this room might help you feel better if you do get upset?

> What might I do to help you if you get upset?

Applying the core principles of trauma-informed practices detailed in the previous pages supports an intervention environment that is trauma-informed. Children must know they are safe—that all they say and all they do is safe from being used to ridicule, belittle, shame, or bully them. The intervention process must be predictable and resources and activities must be identified and readily available to help children deactivate when needed. The environment must be culturally sensitive and the people in it trauma-informed so their interactions and responses to children in that environment are supportive, protective, and reassuring.

Promoting Posttraumatic Growth (PTG) and Resilience

SITCAP is a strength-based, resilience-focused intervention. It directs itself to helping traumatized children (a) change their view of self from victim to survivor, (b) discover that they have the inner resources to heal, and (c) realize the value of others in their efforts to survive. It helps children focus on their strengths and all the parts that make them who they are, and reinforces these aspects through cognitively reframing their thoughts about self, others, and life. In Chapter 9 we discuss specific characteristics that reflect PTG and resilience and activities that help support each.

Summary

In these first three chapters, we have identified the trauma-informed principles in the *SITCAP* process and presented evidence-based research of its value that is also supported by its practice-based history. Having set this foundation, the subsequent chapters discuss in detail the intervention process. Activities are illustrated through case studies, and the most frequently asked questions about the process are answered. We begin the next chapter by discussing the details of our structured drawing activities. Following this discussion, several case examples illustrate that when we move into children's worlds and see what they see, we discover what matters most to them.

Four

Structured Drawing Activities

Beginning with this chapter and throughout the remaining chapters, we provide extensive details regarding *SITCAP (Structured Sensory Interventions for Traumatized Children, Adolescents and Parents)* processes and practices. These are presented as we present them when training professionals. In this chapter we begin by comparing *SITCAP* to the ethnographic interview process used by sociologists, social workers, community psychologists, and businesses to help determine what matters most to those in these varied environments. We compare the value, similarities, and limitations of the ethnographic interview process with the *SITCAP* process. This comparison produces the rationale for the structured drawing practices presented in this chapter. The remainder of the chapter is devoted to our structured drawing practices, including what they accomplish, how they are used, and the practitioner's role in the drawing process. Case examples and illustrations take us into the worlds of grieving and traumatized children while also reinforcing for children the value of their drawings and their efforts to make us understand what matters most to them within the context of their worlds.

Seeing What Children See: The Meaning They Give to Their Experiences

When we come to know traumatized children within the context of their environments and experiences, we can better appreciate what matters most to them and the meaning they give to their experiences, which subsequently drives their behavior. The *SITCAP* process demands that practitioners remain curious in their interactions with children, so they better understand from a qualitative perspective the meaning children give to their experiences. This process is similar to the ethnographic interview. Established many years ago, the ethnographic interview is a qualitative process designed to learn about and understand cultural aspects, which reflect the meanings that guide the life of that culture. Pioneered in the field of sociocultural anthropology (Philipsen, 1992), the process has since been adapted by other disciplines, including social work.

The process is of value because it illuminates the meaning an individual gives to his or her life within the context of his or her experiences and environments. Just as the ethnographic interview helps assess elements of a culture that shape behaviors within that culture, *SITCAP* assesses those elements of children's experiences that help us shape meaningful interventions and interactions. This meaning—this view of self, others, culture, or environment, and life—is what shapes private logic, which then drives behavior. The process helps define what matters most to children and the reasons they do what they do.

The ethnographic interview process is a valuable assessment tool that allows us to make treatment plans and our relationship with the child far more meaningful. However, the process relies on language, verbal, and cognitive processing skills, which are needed to provide descriptive and meaningful responses to the questions presented in the process. Therefore, this process yields limited results with traumatized children, because they are living and functioning primarily in the right brain, not the left brain, where reason, logic, and language are processed. When structured within a trauma-informed context, drawing has been shown to overcome the limits of verbal interviews while also serving as a meaningful intervention with traumatized children.

Drawing is a recognized treatment modality with children (Golub, 1985; Malchiodi, 1990; Riley, 1997, 2001; Roje, 1995). Gross and Haynes (1998) found in their research that drawing encouraged children to tell more than they would during a solely verbal interview. Research at the School of Creative Arts Therapies at the University of Haifa in Israel also found that drawing enhances emotional verbalization among traumatized children compared to verbal interviews alone. In their research, when children in one group were asked to draw first, they included more feelings and sensations and were more descriptive of what happened to them than children in the other group who were asked to only talk about what happened to them (Science 20, 2009).

The *SITCAP* program uses drawing to access the sensations and iconic and implicit trauma memories stored in the right brain. It does this within a structured format that helps children bring us into their world to see what they see when they look at themselves, others, their environment, and life, and the meaning they give to their experiences, so we can appreciate what matters most to them within the context of their experiences. It accomplishes what the ethnographic approach is designed to accomplish, but in our experience with traumatized children, this approach gives us a much more comprehensive view of the child than question-and-answer interviewing and history gathering.

In *SITCAP*'s structured process, drawing is also used to help children find relief from the terror of their experiences and reframe them as well as their view of self and others, in ways that allow them to better manage their memories and regulate the reactions triggered by those memories. *SITCAP*'s structured drawing process not only allows children to give meaning to their lives within the context of their experiences, but it also serves as a trauma-informed, structured intervention process that evidence-based research has clearly shown helps to significantly reduce trauma symptoms and related mental health reactions while improving children's resilience (Raider, Steele, & Kuban, 2012).

Magical Moment

I was with a 9-year-old who was in the middle of working on the sensory theme of anger. Upon entering the room for his session, he announced, "I need to draw and I need to draw right now." Without talking, I provided him with pencils and paper, and he promptly sat down to draw. His finished drawing was of a scene that he had in his head, a trauma memory that had been making him angry and that surfaced between sessions, but that he felt unable to manage outside of the safety of the room. He shoved the paper toward me and said, "Okay, now ask me the questions." I clarified by asking, "Which questions?" He stated, "You know, the ones that help me get my memories out." We proceeded with the questions, he visibly relaxed, and then he high-fived me out the door and said, "I'll be back next week."

Cherie L. Spehar, LCSW, CTS, CTC, Smiling Spirit Pathways, Apex, North Carolina

Todd's Drawing: Giving Meaning to How He Is Experiencing Life

When introduced to *SITCAP*, Todd, age 16, found drawing to be a medium with which he could express what he had no words to describe. Todd's verbal skills were limited. It was difficult for him to identify and verbally express the subjective experiences of his traumatic childhood. He was able to provide details of what happened but not his subjective view of self, others, and life as a result of those experiences. Todd's history of abuse began early in his home with those he trusted. After being removed from his home, he was in and out of multiple foster care homes. At age 16, Todd had consensual sex with a minor, whose parents wanted him prosecuted. He was tried as an adult and incarcerated with the adult population. Left unguarded, he was raped multiple times before he was removed from prison and placed in residential care. Todd had been given several diagnoses, which is so often the case with abused and traumatized children. He was described as impulsive, aggressive, undersocialized, constantly vigilant, and untrusting. At night he would gather all of his belongings around him just in case he had to run. His drawing gives more meaning to how he is experiencing life than was captured or described in his case files.

Putting the Experience in a Contextual Form

In today's world of videogames, the Internet, television, and futuristic movies, children are exposed to far more visual content than in years past. This provides them with a rich library of symbolic images they can use in drawings to more easily communicate how they are experiencing their lives. Feeling overwhelmed and powerless to fight off "the

Figure 4.1   The weight of the world

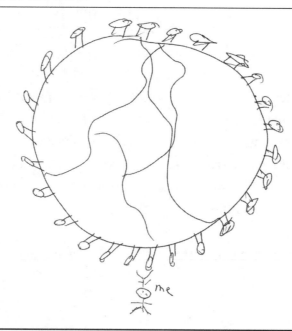

weight of the world" is sometimes depicted in their drawings. How they depict and describe their world can reflect the size, scope, and intensity of their experience.

Todd was asked to draw a picture that would best reflect his anger about all that had happened in his life. Figure 4.1 depicts Todd holding the weight of the world on his shoulders. Most important was the meaning he gave to his *world*. He drew bombs around the earth with wavy lines going through its center. He then indicated that his world was "getting ready to crack." Very few, if any, assessment tools would capture qualitatively the size, weight, and urgency he was feeling in terms of no longer being able to continue his struggle.

We discussed earlier that traumatic experiences are stored implicitly and iconically, without language or context. Drawing provides the opportunity for children to externalize those iconic meanings into a contextual format that makes it easier to then give them meaning and, as we will see, reorder those memories in ways that can be managed.

Accessing, Externalizing, and Concretizing Implicit Memories

In *SITCAP*'s intervention, drawing is used with all ages, including adults. Drawing within this structured process accesses and then externalizes the iconic, implicit memories and meanings of a child's traumatic experiences. Le Bron was referred for depression, had little interest in making friends, was extremely withdrawn, and, at the time of referral, was being bullied by his peers. He no longer had any interest in playing baseball or watching it on television, which was one of his favorite things to do. Le Bron was

8 years old when his father died of a heart attack while watching him play T-ball. At no time did Le Bron ever verbally indicate that he felt responsible for his father's death, until two years later while he was in the *SITCAP* group program *I Feel Better Now!* He was asked to draw a picture of what happened and tell a story about it. When his mother and aunt, who were now raising him, heard his story and the meaning he gave to what happened, they were in disbelief.

Figure 4.2 is Le Bron's simple drawing of what happened the day his father died. Remember that, in the *SITCAP* process, the only validity of what a drawing represents is the meaning the child gives to the drawing. Le Bron's drawing gives no indication as to how it is tied to his depression and avoidant behaviors. However, because his iconic memory is now put into a concrete form, Le Bron can relay the meaning of his drawing to us.

Figure 4.2   A father's death

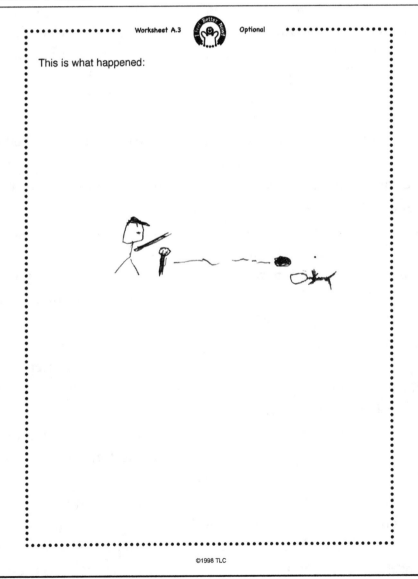

Worksheet A.3   Optional

This is what happened:

©1998 TLC

The drawing shows Le Bron at the tee ready to hit the ball. His father is lying on the ground by first base. When asked what was happening before his father was on the ground, Le Bron indicated he had just hit the ball hard, but it went by his father, who bent down to pick it up and that's when he died. He then said, "If I didn't hit the ball to him he wouldn't have died." The depression he was experiencing since his father's death was understood by everyone, but at no time did family members understand how Le Bron thought he was responsible for this death. His guilt had intensified since then, further complicating his efforts to cope with his father's death. It also left him vulnerable to bullying as a result of the meaning he gave to what happened: *It was my fault, I am bad, punish me.*

Drawing accomplishes what talk alone cannot accomplish. In Le Bron's situation, his behavior was misunderstood, and as a result he received inappropriate attention from the adults in his world. Although Le Bron perceived his actions to be the cause of his father's death, he was unable to find the words to safely express his sense of guilt. This is not unusual, because often the pain of shame accompanies guilt, making what happened too unbearable to talk about. Drawing can be a much safer vehicle for children to express what talk alone cannot express.

Drawing facilitates the following:

➤ Actively involves children in their own healing process, which in turn supports their inner resilience to bounce back from other challenges
➤ Permits children to express what they cannot find the words to describe while they remain internalized in their iconic forms
➤ Permits children to externalize those iconic memories, sensations, and feelings into a concrete, contextual form
➤ Places the trauma into a concrete, manageable container (an 811 piece of paper)
➤ Permits children to experience power over their trauma, which is now something tangible and contained
➤ Permits placing those iconic, implicit memories, sensations, and feelings on a sheet of paper where they can be contained, which allows children to change or add to those memories and do whatever needs to be done with or to them in order to reframe them in ways they can now manage
➤ Facilitates relief from the anxiety, worry, and other trauma-related reactions, because now—externalized into a concrete, tangible form and placed within a container—they can be more easily regulated
➤ Permits children to more easily develop their narrative and give meaning to all of the different aspects of their experiences (Unique to *SITCAP* are the trauma-specific questions that allow children to separately address the common subjective experiences of trauma while shaping their own life narrative as they are living it. At no time

in this process do we ask leading questions, question children's reality, or correct their memory of what happened.)

➤ Provides the practitioner with the opportunity to see the world of grieving and traumatized children as they now see it—their view of self, others, and what matters most to them

➤ Permits children of diverse cultures to express what we have come to know as the common, universal, subjective experiences of trauma despite language and cultural differences

Drawing and Diversity

Children in different parts of the world often portray violence and terror in similar ways. Figures 4.3 and 4.4, for example, are very similar, yet represent very different incidents in different countries with 10 years' difference between the times when these incidents occurred. Figure 4.3 reflects the common themes and symbols that Kuwaiti children depicted during the Gulf War when we visited with them in 1992. At the time, there were still episodes of kidnappings and killings by Iraqi insurgents sneaking into the country, so those occurrences kept the children's fears alive. Figure 4.4 reflects the ways children depicted the 9/11 attack on America years later. The similarities are remarkable, yet not surprising, as we know that subjective experiences can be portrayed using very similar symbols in ways that language prohibits. As we become actual witnesses to the children's views, regardless of how they are symbolically presented, we can better appreciate and help children gain access to or achieve what matters most to them and their efforts to heal.

Figure 4.3   The Gulf War

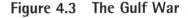

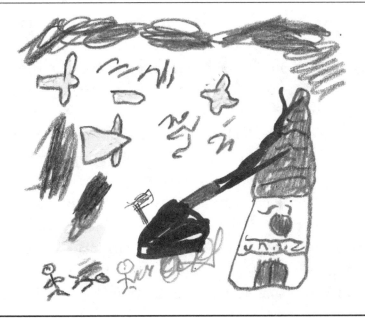

Figure 4.4   9/11 attack on America

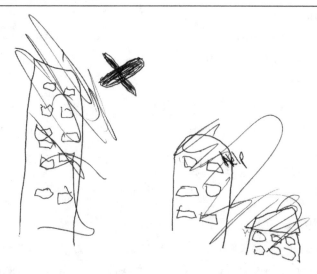

How Children Draw Does Not Matter

How children draw their traumatized memories simply does not matter in the *SITCAP* process, because drawings are not used for evaluation or assessment purposes of any kind. Furthermore the practitioner's role in this process is not to interpret, analyze, or pass judgment on children's drawings. The practitioner's role is to remain curious and present so children have the opportunity to develop their own stories and descriptions of how each of the details in their drawings fit into their overall trauma experiences.

It is not at all unusual for a simplistic drawing to represent a significant part of an experience. Figure 4.5 is a drawing by Steven, a 14-year-old, who was born to an addicted mother. During the first six years of his life, Steven was in and out of numerous foster care homes. From ages 6 to 14, he lived with an aunt, who abused him until he was removed from her home. His drawing is nondescript, and yet his story reflects the kind of details we often hear described by children in domestic violence and substance-abusing family situations.

Steven, like others, initially uses nondescriptive symbols rather than a detailed, recognizable picture. He drew the first box, which represents him coming from his aunt's house walking to his mother's house—the larger box. Here he stopped drawing but instead kept his black ink pen steadily coloring in the large image below the larger box. The image did not represent anything in particular according to Steven; he just kept his pen repetitively moving across the paper. His head and eyes remained focused on his drawing as he was asked trauma-specific questions to help him tell his story. In his own way, he was externalizing in symbolic form the implicit memories of his collective

Figure 4.5 Child born to addicted mother

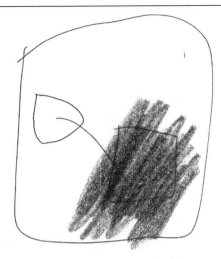

experiences. Following is his story, which also reflects the details that children in violent homes present:

My aunt beat me up again, and I ran from her house. I walked down an alley. It was hot outside. It was summer, the alley smelled like garbage and animals. I saw one of my older brother's friends when I was walking. He looked meaner than ever. When I got to my mother's house, my little sister was in the front room on the couch crying. I heard my mother and brother arguing in the kitchen. I know my mom was high. My brother was yelling and beating my mother. I took my sister into the front bedroom 'cause she didn't need to see this, and I told her I'd be right back. When I got to the kitchen, my brother was hitting my mother with a plate over her head, and then he had a fork at her throat. My mother fell to the floor, and my brother kicked her in the head. I pulled him away from her and beat him in the face until I knocked him out. My mother started foaming at the mouth when I called 911. She even peed in her pants right there on the kitchen floor. I thought she was dying. The police and ambulance came and the police took my brother. I held my sister and we followed the ambulance. We were in the backseat of another cop car.

At this point he began sobbing. This child's drawing was very nondescript, and yet it represented a significant part of his overall experience, which later gave meaning to his aggressive, assaultive behavior. It also demonstrated that he could initiate a reciprocal relationship, as documented by his sensitivity to the impact this incident was having on his sister and his ability to protect her emotionally and physically at the time.

Figure 4.6   Eleven-year-old brother

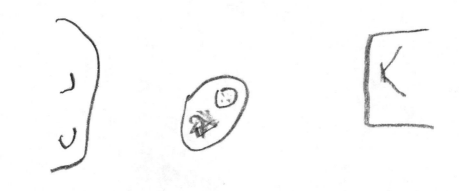

Figure 4.7   Six-year-old sister

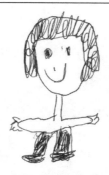

Figure 4.6 is a drawing by Peter, an 11-year-old boy whose stepsister was sexually assaulted and murdered. Figure 4.7 is the drawing of Emma, his 6-year-old sister. Her drawing is far more dimensional than her brother's; however, what children draw does not matter—what matters is the meaning children give to the drawing. Peter's description of what he had drawn was as meaningful as the more-dimensional drawing of his younger sister. Emma's drawing contains full-body figures. The brother draws "C" for his step sister and "L" for her boyfriend. His story about "C" and "L" is as insightful as his younger sister's story related to the full figure in her drawing.

Pursuing Details Matters

Details are very important. In this process, we take the position that whatever children draw, they expect us to be curious about every aspect, every line, scribble, shaded area, figure, and object. Any one of these elements could contain the core element of their experience that shaped their private logic and is driving their behavior. Figure 4.8 is a drawing by Erica, a 16-year-old who endured repeated sexual assaults. The mother pressed charges against the live-in relative, and shortly thereafter he killed himself. There

Figure 4.8   Repeated sexual assault

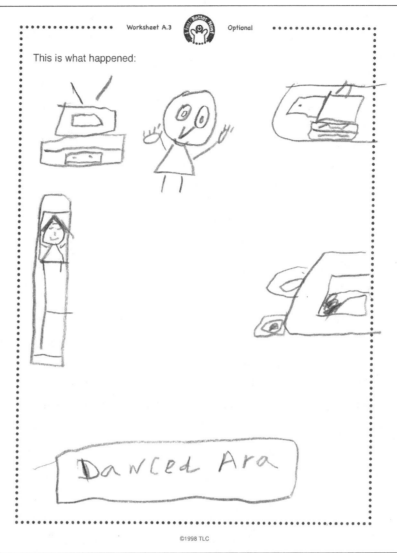

are two specific elements in her drawing that represent two different parts of her story. Had these elements not been asked about, it would have significantly lessened our appreciation of what was fueling her arousal and what mattered most to her. It also depicts how some children in violent homes find a way to create a safe place for themselves while trapped in that environment.

In the upper center of the drawing is a picture of her abuser. Erica told how he repeatedly abused her in the basement room where she stayed. However, had she not been asked about the detail of her drawing of her abuser, we would never have understood its relationship with her behavior. Specifically, she was asked, "Tell me about his eyes." Her response was, "I feel like he is always watching me." The ongoing persistence of arousal is now explained by the ongoing intrusiveness of her abuser's gaze.

At the bottom of the page she drew a separate area that she identified as her dance area. This was significant because this is where she would come when her abuser was not around. She would play her music as loudly as she could and dance to the music for as long as she could. This became her safe place, her self-regulating activity that buffered the terror she felt every night when it was time to sleep. Within a trauma-informed framework, music and dance became resources of resilience and self-regulation that can now become an integral part of her treatment plan. Her story teaches us as practitioners that we can help children who are trapped in violent and unhealthy environments by helping them create a safe place—a place that momentarily allows them some relief, a time to regulate/deactivate the aroused state they are forced to live in because of the constant anticipation of being traumatized.

Beginning the Process

The use of drawing in the *SITCAP* process is only initiated after the education phase, in which children are introduced to what trauma is and what it can do to us. Children's reactions are also normalized, and they are given an explanation as to how the intervention works, what they will be asked to do, and how they can say *yes* or *no* to anything they are asked to do or talk about. If available, it helps to show simplistic examples of what other children have drawn while explaining it does not matter how or what the child draws. This session also includes administering any pretest evaluations that are deemed appropriate. A previous intake session is held with parents or guardians to gather their observations and understanding of what they believe is happening with their children, to tell them how the process works, and to discuss the role they can play in supporting their children by attending the session when it comes time for their children to tell their stories to them. Once this process is completed, the drawing process begins. Children are asked in the first or second session to draw a picture of what happened so they can tell us a story about it. There are several possible responses to what children draw.

Possible Responses

Sometimes what children draw has nothing to do with what happened, but this is where they feel safe starting. This generally occurs with children under the age of 8. However, even younger children will sometimes draw what happened when they are asked. The cornerstone of all trauma-informed care is safety. If what children draw has nothing to do with what happened, simply ask them to tell their story. Allow them to tell the complete story, because this is where they feel safe beginning. When they are finished, they can be redirected by asking, "What I would like you to do now is draw a picture of what happened when. . . . "

For some children, a drawing may contain multiple elements of their experience that will take an entire session for them to describe. Occasionally one of those elements may lead us to ask them to draw another picture related to that element, because it has its own story and is important to their overall experience. However, additional drawings are only initiated when the story associated with the original drawing is completed, so as to leave children in control of the direction they need to take us in.

For other children, a drawing may contain only one aspect of the overall experience, and children only spend a few minutes describing that part of their experience. In this situation, we simply move into the structured, sequential activities related to the major experiences of trauma, allowing them to build their story one activity at a time. It is important to appreciate that traumatized children may need time to get to that part of the story that defines them the most, teach us what matters most, and describe the meaning they have given their experiences. Being patient and following the pace children set is sometimes initially difficult for practitioners, especially when what children are presenting does not seem to be making sense. *SITCAP* is structured to take children from the *then* of their experiences to how they are experiencing themselves, others, and their environments *now*. For many children, it takes time to safely bring us into their worlds to see what they now see, feel what they now feel, and think what they now think, in order for us to make sense of their worlds.

A drawing at times represents several different traumatic experiences. Children often separate their individual experiences by drawing a dividing line between those experiences or placing them apart from one another on the paper. Figure 4.9 represents how some children depict the multiple traumas in their lives when they are asked to draw a picture of what happened so they can tell us about it. They create multiple windows or sections and draw an incident in each. When this occurs, children are given the choice of describing each one briefly or selecting the one experience they want us to know about. When children have no more to tell about their drawing, they will generally indicate this by saying "That's it." However, we would, if appropriate, continue presenting those questions related to what we are curious about. When they are no longer responding, we simply ask if there is anything else they want us to know and, if not, then move to the next activity.

Note Taking

Notes are not taken during this process. Taking notes not only distracts children but also impedes our efforts to remain curious. Note taking may create anxiety for many children, especially those who have been involved with child protective services and juvenile justice. They will worry about our letting others read those notes and what we write about them. The importance of what children reveal, the meaning they give their experience, and their view of self and others is not likely to be forgotten and can be easily summarized after the session. We also encourage and caution practitioners about being too detailed with file notes. The caution is real, because files can be subpoenaed and the information can be misinterpreted or misused.

Figure 4.9   Multiple traumas

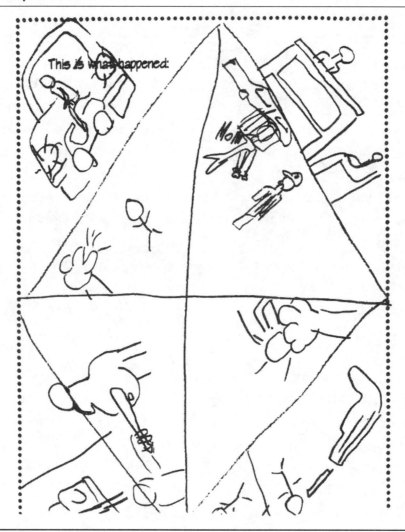

When drawings are subpoenaed, it is very important to repeatedly indicate that the drawing process was not used for evaluation purposes of any kind, and therefore you cannot interpret what any aspect or element of the drawing infers, only what that child indicated it represented. You are not likely to remember all of the different components of the child's story, only his or her overall story. When we begin to infer what parts of a drawing reflect about the child's psyche, we are entering very dangerous territory that even well-trained forensic specialists navigate with great caution. Remember, the only meaning children's drawings have are the meanings they assign to them.

What We Do With Drawings

We do not send children home with their drawings until the final session and, even then, only if children and their parents or guardians have participated in the joint session when the children use their drawings to tell their stories to their parents or guardians. This is usually

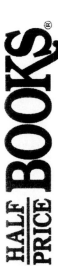

HALF PRICE BOOKS®

Half Price Books
3860 LA REUNION PKWY
DALLAS, TX 75212
OFS OrderID 11335724

Thanks for your order! Your order number is R154643571

We hope you love it, but just in case something isn't perfect, or if you need to manage your other orders, please visit HPB.com/user/orders. Or, contact our Customer Care team at customercare@hpb.com or call 800.883.2114 Mon – Fri, 8 a.m. – 7 p. m. and Sat-Sun 8 a.m. – 4 p.m. Central.

Visit our stores to sell your books, music, movies games for cash.

SKU	ISBN/UPC	Title & Author/Artist	Shelf ID	Qty
S273833250	9781118543177	Working With Grieving and Traumatized Chil... Steele William/ Kuban, Caelan / Steele, W....	08--03--5	1

SHIPPED EXPEDITED TO
Adrienne Kapocius
5015 Guaine Ct
Fort Wayne Indiana 46815

ORDER# R154643571
HPB.com

completed in the seventh session. This joint session is preceded by a brief session and/or phone conversation with parents to explain why this process is critical to their children's well-being and to discuss ways they can best respond to their children and the drawings.

Before the child–parent session, practitioners must prepare children for telling their stories using their drawings. It is very important to ask whether there are any drawings they do not want their parents or guardians to see. These are removed to maintain trust in us and to protect the children, as well as to follow their intuitive sense and experience as to what will keep them safe from negative and/or critical responses from their parents.

We do not write on children's drawings. Their drawings are their life—a very big part of their life. Writing on drawings breaches the boundaries of respect and trust established by this process. Copies of drawings can be used for written references, but remember to heed the caution just expressed regarding note taking.

At the very last session, it is important to lay all of the drawings out on a table so we can review with the child all of the different parts of that child's varied experiences. It is essential to ask the following: "As you look at all of your drawings, all of the different parts of your story, is there anything you wish to change, anything or anyone you wish to add? If so, go ahead and add or make that change now." Not to ask children to do this is to cheat them of the opportunity to reorder their stories in a way they can best manage and to reveal what may matter most to them. At the same time, if there are any parts of the drawings we did not ask about previously, it is important to ask about them at this point, because they may contain the most meaningful part of the child's experience. More than once we have learned how one previously missed query, when revisited, can significantly alter our view of children and their views of themselves and their lives.

Drawing Activities

Following are eight examples of the drawing activities in *SITCAP*. They do differ slightly between children and adolescents. The sequence of activities will also be different between the two age ranges. The graphics used in each activity will differ as well, in order to accommodate developmental differences. For example, the worry activity, which asks children to show how small or big their worry is at the time, uses different-sized animals for children younger than 6 years of age. They color the animal that best shows the size of their worry. For children in the 6- to 12-year range, different-sized squares are used. They fill in the square that best reflects the size of their worry. For adolescents and adults, stick figures carrying rocks of different sizes that weigh them down are used to depict the size and weight of their worry.

Each drawing activity is preceded by a series of curious, open questions, or in some cases other activities that bring children to other specific drawing tasks. Any one drawing can lead to another drawing as a natural way for children to continue to elaborate on elements of their experiences. This is not an all-inclusive listing of the drawing activities, but it does highlight a number of the specific subjective experiences of children that are addressed in the program:

> This is me _____. I was ____ years old when ____.
>
> Draw me a picture of what happened.
>
> Fill in the box that shows how small or big your worry is for you now. (This activity is repeated at the completion of intervention to show the reduction of the child's worry following intervention.)
>
> Draw me a picture of what your anger looks like.
>
> Draw me a picture of what your hurt or fear looks like.
>
> Draw me a picture of what ___ looked like when it happened or, if this is about the child him- or herself, draw me a picture of what you looked like at the time this happened.
>
> Draw me a picture of the person or thing that caused this to happen.
>
> Draw me a picture of what you would like to see happen to the person or thing that caused this to happen.

Point of Interest

Nightmares

Nightmares are typically more common in children than in adults. One in every four children experiences at least one nightmare per week, and as many as 50% of these children have nightmares significant enough in frequency and intensity to cause parents to be concerned (Schedl, 2010). Nightmares that follow traumatic life events are typically experienced in the form of a recurrent nightmare that graphically and specifically reenacts their traumatic experience. These nightmares can occur repeatedly in any given sleep period or may persist for decades after the actual event has occurred. Common reactions upon waking from a nightmare include increased heart and respiratory rates, sweating, sharpened attention, fear, anger, panic, or feeling helpless or out of control. Adverse reactions to nightmares can subside quickly, but for some children, the reactions can persist for hours, days, or even weeks.

Working with nightmares to facilitate reduction in frequency and intensity is possible in a safe and structured setting. The goal is to allow the person who is experiencing nightmares to explore the content while helping them maintain a sense of control. Helping the person gradually disclose difficult content and checking in with them frequently to assess their level of arousal can accomplish this goal. The integration of relaxation techniques, such as positive imagery, may be necessary during intervention. Ultimately, you want to shift the person from feeling stuck in their nightmare. One way to do this is to ask questions like, "If you could rewrite the nightmare, how would you rewrite it?" or "If you could change the ending of the nightmare, tell me what that would be like." Taking this one step further and asking them to draw how their ideal ending would look may allow for some additional relief, as it makes the person an active participant in their healing, while moving the nightmare outside of themselves into a concrete form with which they can do whatever they need to do to no longer be frightened by it.

When a Story Triggers Another Drawing

There are additional drawing activities often driven by children's stories. As indicated earlier, any one drawing can lead to the need for additional drawings, such as asking children to draw a picture of their family doing something. Children may draw a small stick figure with little or no facial detail. They could later be asked for greater detail by having them take another sheet of paper and using the whole sheet of paper to draw a picture of what that person's face looks like. This gives us a closer look and generally leads to more detailed information about that person, their relationship, and some aspect of the trauma that was not previously revealed. Another example is when children draw a picture of themselves. They will be asked, "Is this a picture of you now or then?" Depending on the answer, they are asked later to draw another picture of themselves as they were then or are now so we might visually see how they now define themselves and their world.

In many ways, drawing accomplishes what formal assessments do not, by putting children's behaviors, thoughts, and affect within a context that, from a trauma-informed perspective, helps makes sense of their lives as well as reveal the qualitative experiences they may need to strengthen their resilience—not just diminish their symptoms. Most important drawing it more clearly defines what matters most to children in ways that often mean more to the practitioner than descriptions given from test results.

Summary

In this chapter we mentioned the use of trauma-specific questions to help children bring us into their worlds and help us remain curious so we can be more of a witness than a clinician. In the next chapter we identify these questions and how they are used, and we discuss the critical role being curious plays in our intervention process. We illustrate, as we do in our actual trainings, how we become that curious practitioner and the lessons learned by being curious rather than analytical. We conclude by identifying the four criteria used to develop cognitive reframing statements that are personalized to children's unique experiences in ways that they can be accepted and internalized by the children.

CHAPTER Five

Curiosity and the Trauma Questioning Process

In this chapter we discuss the value of curiosity as a treatment process, followed by *SITCAP*'s process of trauma-specific questioning. This process is designed to keep us in the role of being curious, as well as to give children multiple ways to portray, describe, and communicate how they are experiencing the very facets of their past and current experiences. We also describe in detail several activities used in our trauma certification training that help practitioners break old *mindsets* to become nonknowing, curious practitioners versus clinicians who analyze and try to make sense out of everything they learn about children. We hesitate placing this at the beginning of this chapter, because the process is not about having a list of questions and then going down the list asking one question after another. Instead, in this process, children lead the intervention, allowing us to know when to pursue these questions. This process helps prevent our intrusive interruptions of children's descriptions while they bring us deeper into their life experiences. Therefore, we begin by discussing the value of curiosity and its role in creating pathways for us to build relationships with children that are empathetic, attuned, and in sync with how they are experiencing their worlds.

Curiosity

We discuss the value of curiosity because, without curiosity, we would never learn and others would never benefit from what we learn by being curious. In treatment, curiosity is a teacher for both the person being curious as well as the one responding to our curiosity.

In the *SITCAP* process, curiosity drives the critical healing journey of children. The book *Clinical Values and Emotions That Guide Psychoanalytic Treatment* (Beuchler, 2004) emphasizes at the very beginning of the first chapter how curiosity about the unfamiliar is a motivating factor in the therapeutic progress. In writing about therapists who are too confident with where they are going, Padesky (1993) states, "(They) only look ahead and miss a detour that can lead to a better place."

Asking "What" Not "Why"

By asking *what* rather than *why*, we remain witnesses to children's experiences rather than analytical interpreters of their experiences. In the previous chapter, we indicated that the only validity to the meaning of children's drawings is the meaning the children give them—that is their reality. Their reality, as they are living it, drives their behaviors. To focus on trying to answer why children are the way they are keeps us leading the intervention and prevents us from discovering how they actually experience themselves, their environments, and their worlds, all of which are the driving forces behind their behaviors. Because traumatized children are living in and responding from their lower survival brain and limbic systems rather than from their cortical, cognitive brain, the analytical and reasoning *why* approach simply does not match the way traumatized children are processing their day-to-day experiences (Gil, 2006; Levine & Kline, 2007; Steele & Malchiodi, 2012; Stien & Kendall, 2004). By being curious, we discover how children view and react to their daily environments.

Curiosity: The Cornerstone of Empathy

Being curious also allows practitioners to begin to establish an empathetic relationship between children and themselves in the very first session. Curiosity is the cornerstone of empathy. Empathy is established by creating an atmosphere in which children tell us about (or reveal via drawing) their experiences in enough concrete detail that we feel the emotions (Smith, 2012). Curiosity creates this atmosphere and encourages children to give such detail.

Furthermore, by remaining curious, we remain in sync with traumatized children. Neuroscientist Ramachandran (2011) talks about the importance of *mirror neurons*, and how they are one of the most exciting discoveries in recent years. Mirror neurons refer to brain cells that are triggered when we are in action and when we are watching others in action. They allow us to know what others are feeling. Putting ourselves in the role of being a witness, seeing what children see when they look at themselves and us, is really what provides insight into their worlds—or what Siegel (2003) refers to as *mind sight*, knowing what another feels. Perry (2009) refers to this process as *attunement*, or being present and in sync with traumatized children. From a developmental view, we are not passive participants in our own development, but we are continually responding to our environment and those in our environment. In essence, we develop as a result of the interactions we experience within our varied environments and how others respond to us. This is referred to as *reciprocal interaction* (Sohn & Grayson, 2005). By being curious and willing to allow children to lead us into their worlds, our interaction is experienced as less of a threat. Once this interaction is established, children reciprocate by becoming curious about our view and what else we might be curious about as we become attuned and in sync with each other.

Giving Children the Lead

The additional value derived from being curious, being the nonknowing practitioner, is that it allows children to lead the intervention (Condy & Kehman, 2007). Henrikson (2012) wrote:

> In a collaborative language system approach the therapist maintains his stance of not knowing and one that is curious. The therapist is not assuming that he or she knows what is best. And the therapist makes every effort to be curious about and learn about the client's objective reality and worldview because this is the subjective reality in which the presenting problems exist.

The reality is we cannot understand children's subjective experiences until we know them like they know them. We need to know what the experiences of children have been like for them and the meaning they give to these experiences, because that meaning drives their behavior. Only by being curious and having them externalize their experiences into drawings are we able to witness these experiences as they live them.

John Seita was 7 years old when he was placed in his first foster care home. Over the next 11 years, he would be in and out of 15 different foster care homes. He learned not to trust anyone during that time and engaged in the primary survival-driven behaviors seen so often in traumatized youth: aggressive, assaultive, oppositional, defiant, impulsive, and unpredictable behavior. Now a university professor at the School of Social Work, Michigan State University, he has become a very strong and active advocate of foster care reform. His turnaround was a result of the time he spent at Starr Commonwealth, the home of TLC.

We mention John's story because Starr Commonwealth focuses primarily on being *attuned* to children while providing them, over time, with opportunities to redefine their self by exposing them to a myriad of new experiences and relationships with those who remain curious and attuned. Seita said of this life-changing experience:

> It is clear to me by way of time and the wisdom of personal and professional hindsight, that only once I found myself in a safe, structured and caring environment where others took the time to connect with me by being consistently patient, but also curious as to what I thought, what I believed, how I looked at myself as well as what I saw in those trying to help me, did my mistrust fade and my trauma ebb away. (Steele & Malchiodi, 2012, p. 155)

Hughes (2009) wrote:

> When curiosity is directed toward the child's experience rather than toward the factual events in his life and when it is conveyed with both affective and reflective

features, the child is likely to go with the therapist very deeply into his or her life story and experience a co-regulating of emotions related to what is being explored and the meaning given those events. (p. 169)

We have described how *SITCAP* is a structured process, a safe process, and a curious process that allows children to communicate more than they can in direct verbal interviewing processes. We have addressed how structured drawing activities can help bring us into the world of children as witnesses, seeing what they see—their view of self, others, and life. The *SITCAP* process contains the essential elements that Dr. Seita attributed to the transforming of his life and that Perry, Seigel, Padesky, Beuchler, and Henrikson cited as critical to therapeutic progress, all of which are derived from being curious within the structured process of *SITCAP*. The trauma-specific questions and process we have developed support our ability to remain curious.

Trauma-Specific Questioning

Unique to *SITCAP* is the use of its trauma-specific questioning process that allows us to:

➤ Frame our relationship with children as a curious one
➤ Remain patient
➤ Follow the pace children set while walking hand-in-hand with the children in sync, in their world
➤ Introduce children to new ways to view themselves and their lives
➤ Provide them with the opportunity to redefine themselves within the context of this safe and curious relationship

Our trauma-specific questions are designed to address what TLC has identified as the most common subjective experiences of trauma: terror, worry, hurt, anger, revenge, accountability (guilt and shame), feeling unsafe, powerless, and engaging in victim thinking. They are also designed to help children:

➤ Explore the details of their experiences in a variety of ways
➤ Discover how to best externalize, portray, or present their experiences in ways that are meaningful for them, even when words are not available to describe them
➤ Arrive at a new view of themselves, others, and life that reflects the self as a resilient survivor

SITCAP's trauma-specific questioning is also a process designed to help children discover multiple ways to communicate in detail:

➤ The elements of their traumatic experiences
➤ How they experienced these traumatic elements

> What made them think and do or not think and not do
> How these experiences shaped their self-image, private logic, and current view of self, others, and life, all of which drive behavior

The questions are initiated following specific activities that focus on one of the common reactions of trauma, such as fear or hurt. At all times children lead the focus of that session while the questions are in response to the descriptions or story they are telling at the time. The questions are integrated with the activities to help them also *end* the story of their past life in a way they can manage while beginning a *new chapter* in their present life. Curious questioning in this process allows us to continually move children from the *then* to the *now* of their view of self and others; once in the *now*, we continue to use curiosity to help them define their view of self in the future.

Being curious, never knowing where children are going to take us, can initially "stump" practitioners whose mindset is to attempt to figure things out, to formulate insightful responses to children in the hope that they will agree and see things from our perspective. This approach often makes very little sense to children, because what may be true may not be of value based on their implicit view of themselves and others at the time. Because they are living and processing day-to-day life experiences in their *sensory* brain, truth has limited impact on change.

Furthermore, *SITCAP*'s questioning process allows children's implicit memories to be safely externalized into a concrete form, given a context in which they can give those implicit memories and experiences a new meaning. In this process, children experience relief, while the practitioner remains curious. Using *SITCAP* activities and integrating its trauma-specific questions with the drawing process helps children redefine their view of self in the future with strength and resilience.

The Process: Experiencing the Lessons Being Learned

In our training we reach a point when it's time to ask practitioners to apply what they have learned. They are presented with a series of drawings and must respond to what they are curious about when looking at these drawings. Often they do not hear the references the child—in this case, the trainer—gives them to pursue, because they're trying too hard to figure out what the drawing means. Old mindsets make it difficult for them to be curious. Usually by the time the fifth drawing is presented, this old mindset has been broken, and they begin to respond with natural curiosity to the details of the drawings and the references they are given to pursue. They begin following rather than trying to stay one step ahead of the child.

We walk you through this activity as it is presented and processed in training. This will further demonstrate what we mean by being curious and allowing children to lead the session. Once we have given more attention to this process, we provide a listing of some of the trauma-specific questions used to address specific subjective experiences of trauma. If children's descriptions or stories do not present an opportunity to use these questions, only then do we take the lead and use the questions to focus on a specific subjective experience. If children, for example, do not communicate the worries that have resulted from their experience, then we initiate a focus on worry using activities that also allow for the use of questions specific to that reaction. In essence, we want the process to be as natural and spontaneous as possible, rather than being experienced as intrusive.

The activity begins by informing participants that once the drawing is presented, we will simply go around the room and ask each participant what they are curious about. Keep in mind that their curiosity will generate from the trainer, who gives responses similar to responses that children have given to such drawings. This new information or the references given to them will allow them to follow and expand on what to pursue with continued curiosity. They are told they will be presented with several drawings and go through the same process with each drawing and, as a result, find themselves becoming more curious practitioners.

Figure 5.1 is the first drawing presented. As we select participants for their questions, we usually hear, "Who is this person?" and "How do you know this person?" At this point, the old mindset wins out. The two next questions we most often hear are, "Why is one eye different than the other?" and "What is he smiling about?" Using the word *why* lets us know that practitioners are slipping into more of an analytical approach and that they are assuming the difference in the ways the eyes are drawn has some psychological meaning. The trainer responds to this question by saying, "I don't know" or "That's just the way I drew it." He may also just shrug his shoulders as if to say "I don't know" or "I can't tell you." We simply do not ask *why* questions in this process, because the reality is that traumatized children rarely can answer the question "Why?" In the second question, the practitioners are assuming the child is smiling, when the child could in fact be dead or

Figure 5.1   A child's face

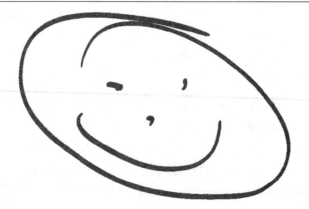

the child who has drawn the face has a different meaning of what that smile represents. Maybe it is not a smile at all.

Lessons Learned

➤ Never assume we know what we are looking at.
➤ The only validity to what is drawn is the meaning children give to their drawings.
➤ It is best to be general in our queries by simply asking, "Can you tell me about the mouth?" or by pointing to that part of the drawing that interests us and saying, "Tell me about this."

We then continue to go around the room and have participants ask what else they might be curious about, but frequently we have to help them get their curiosity restarted, because they see nothing else but the face in the drawing. They forget the reference is not just about a face but a child, and that something is happening or happened to the child. This helps some participants get started, and we hear such questions as:

➤ "What is happening to you (if the child draws himself), your friend, sibling, or to that person?"
➤ "Where were you when this happened?
➤ "Was anyone else there?"
➤ "What else happened?"
➤ "What did you do?"

At this point the curiosity begins to diminish, and we need to again help by asking, "If this is a child, is this what a child looks like? What's missing?" Immediately they respond with, "Where's the rest of the body?"

The one remaining aspect of this drawing is that children exist in an environment. Again, because the drawing is of a child, we can then ask where this is taking place and follow up with questions about what the environment is like; who was there; what sounds, smells, sensations of touch, or visuals remind the child of what happened then; what others were doing at the time; what happened in the days and weeks that followed; and so on.

Lessons Learned

➤ If a child presents a drawing involving a person—regardless of whether it is a stick figure, with or without a body—it gives us permission to ask whatever we are curious about related to getting to know this person in the drawing, his or her relationship to the child, and the meaning of the drawing. Once this is learned, the questions flow: "What else can you tell me about this child? What did he do when this happened? What happened to him? Was anyone else there?"

Figure 5.2   What is this?

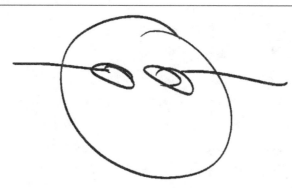

> ➢ If the drawing of the child is the child who's actually doing the drawing, then we simply change the reference and ask the same questions, for example, "What were you doing when this happened?"
> ➢ At times the trauma is not what was happening to the child, but what was happening in the child's environment. Curiosity would just naturally move us to the surrounding environment and all that was happening in that environment, as well as how and what the child experienced in that environment.

We now move to the next drawing, Figure 5.2. Half of the group will assume this is a drawing of a child, but the other half are not sure what to make of it. Those who assume this is a child ask related questions until we pause and indicate that we cannot be sure this is a drawing of a child. This reinforces that the only validity to what a drawing represents is what the child tells us it represents.

We inform them that this is also a drawing of a child, so they can move in the direction of asking more about that child and the different aspects of his drawing. They frequently then begin with, "What are those lines?" referring to the lines at eye level. They learn these lines could represent eyeglasses, the rim of a hat, or a baseball bat that was used to beat the child. As the activity continues, they realize they would engage in the same questions identified in the first lesson, keeping in mind that they would also curiously pursue other references given to them in response to their questions.

In this activity we will insert more specific information as to what is happening to help the participants pursue the stated references with the same curiosity. For example, we might say, "This child was badly beaten and needed to go to the hospital." There are two references or two parts of this experience to pursue: the experience of being beaten and the experience while in the hospital, which in this case was extremely terrifying for the child, who was activated when placed in restraints so he would not make his injuries worse while the doctors tended to him.

Lessons Learned

➤ The best way to begin this questioning process, once a child has completed his drawing, is by stating, "Tell me the story" or "Tell me about your drawing."

➤ One drawing can lead to multiple experiences and other trauma references we want to pursue with similar curiosity.

The next drawing, Figure 5.3, is used to reinforce that it doesn't matter what or how the child draws, but what matters is the meaning he gives to what he draws. When we indicate this too is a child, participants usually respond immediately. We now hear many of the same questions presented in the previous activities and, depending on what the child (trainer) tells them is happening, those references are also pursued with the same curiosity. There is one additional aspect we point out regarding this drawing. We ask, "If this is a child, what are you literally having trouble with as you look at this child?" The usual response is about the drawing being so small they cannot see the child in any detail. This tells us that the practitioners have made much progress with remaining curious and understanding the process.

Lessons Learned

➤ What or how children draw does not matter, but the meaning they give to their drawings is what matters the most.

➤ We use this as an example of how one drawing can lead to another. Presented with this drawing, we would ask the child, "I wonder if you could take another sheet of paper and use that entire sheet to draw yourself (friend, brother, etc.), so I can get a closer look at you (him)." Most children will do this, and it often encourages a child to reveal much more about what is happening because they too are taking a closer look.

The next drawing, Figure 5.4, is a burning house. Participants usually ask a quick dozen questions related to what is happening. However, the one question rarely asked is, "Did anyone die?" We take time to process this, because it reflects the mindset that we must be cautious about what we ask. Our response to this caution is that they need to take themselves out of the therapist/counselor role. We reframe this by saying, "If you

Figure 5.3   What or how a child draws does not matter

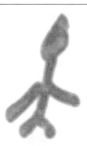

Figure 5.4   A burning home

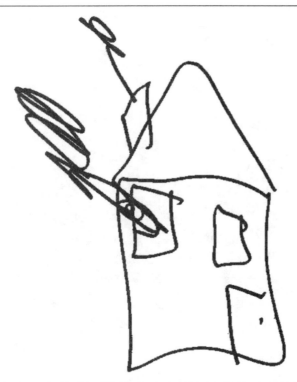

were a friend, and you heard that your friend's house caught on fire, what would be your spontaneous response?" It would likely be "Is my friend okay or did anyone die?" Failing to remain curious about all that could have happened takes us from being in sync and attuned to being detached or outside of the child's world.

The other aspect of this drawing that teaches an additional lesson about the process emerges when we ask them, "As you look at this drawing, where are you in reference to the house?" It takes a moment, but they do understand the question and reply that they are outside of the house.

Lessons Learned

➢ Whatever children draw and whatever references they give us in their descriptions of what is drawn, they fully expect us to be curious about every aspect. By drawing what they draw, they are giving us permission to pursue every element.

➢ If we don't ask about all the aspects of their drawing and the references they give us, they interpret this to mean we are not listening, are making our own decisions about what is and is not important, or that we really are not that interested in their experiences. In either case, they experience a disconnect with us and become less eager to bring us into their lives.

➢ When a child draws about a situation that places us outside of what is happening, we need to go inside, because the trauma reference may actually have taken place inside.

In this example, there are several ways to have the child take us inside his house. One example might be to ask him to draw a picture or tell us what his room was like before the fire. Once in the house, after taking us into his room, the child is then likely to provide numerous references about what life was like in his home. If the child draws a situation in which we are inside, we want to eventually be curious as to what is happening outside of that environment, because again this part of his experience may contain another and/or more trauma-specific reference.

Once we cover all of the curious questions that could be asked about a house fire, we ask participants to then tell us what the next part of the story might be about. Usually someone says that the family may need to go to a temporary shelter. Following the temporary shelter experience, and depending on the damage the fire produced, the family may need to relocate, receive aid, or even become homeless.

Lessons Learned

- We stress that the trauma is not just what happened that day, but all the changes and challenges that had to be endured in the days, weeks, and months that followed.
- We stress that our role of being curious must take us from the *then* of children's experiences to the *now* of their experience to best appreciate how they are now viewing themselves, others, and life.

To further help participants feel comfortable with being curious, we present this final drawing, Figure 5.5. We change the process at this point and instead of asking them what questions they may have about the drawing, we ask them to use their imagination to simply relate what the scribbling in the mouth area could represent. We generally end up with 20 to 30 possibilities. Some of these possibilities include that it represents stitches, braces, sexual assault, physical beating, blood, saying something that should not have been said, secrets, and duct tape. Someone always mentions chocolate, and eventually we hear, "Maybe he didn't like the way he drew it, so he crossed it out."

Figure 5.5   Use your imagination

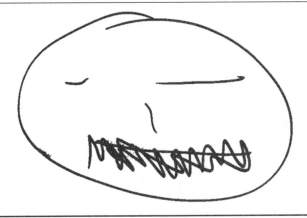

Lessons Learned

> ➤ There are many possible meanings about what a child draws.
> ➤ By activating our imagination about what those possibilities could be, we automatically become more curious about all the aspects of the drawing as well as the possible aspects of all that could have happened.

Questioning the Child's Subjective Experiences

We have mentioned the common subjective experiences of trauma several times: terror, worry, hurt, and so forth. When these experiences or themes emerge in children's descriptions of what is happening or happened in their drawings, we simply expand our curiosity of those themes using the questioning process. However, descriptions given by children will not always address these subjective experiences. Because it is so important to give traumatized children the opportunity to address these subjective experiences, each *SITCAP* session focuses on one of the subjective experiences. In some cases, children will spend a great deal of time bringing us into that experience, and at other times they spend very little time because they have very little to share. Because it is also important for children to externalize the implicit sensory memories, sensations, and affect associated with these experiences, they are introduced in each session to several different activities to help them discover different ways to best present these to us. We will present many of the curious questions that can be asked about two of these subjective experiences to further demonstrate the process, the value of curiosity, and all it accomplishes. The first subjective experience is *hurt*, and the second is the *worst part*.

Hurt

The first theme is hurt. We address hurt as a way to help the child identify how his body is reacting to his traumatic experiences, how he experiences the hurt, what it makes him do and think, and how by externalizing it, making it concrete, and putting it into a container he can begin to regulate that hurt, find relief from it, and diminish its hold on him.

We ask participants to identify in their groups all of the questions that can be asked about hurt. We then go to each group, asking for only one question from each group, but keep returning to each group until all of the questions they have listed about hurt have been asked. This activity helps them discover all the ways they can remain curious and explore one theme or one experience in different ways. We start by presenting the question, "Where did you feel hurt the most in your body?" From here they are given time in their groups to identify additional questions to ask about hurt. Depending on the group size, we can identify 30 to 40 different questions. Following is a listing of some of those questions:

➤ Is the hurt still there?

➤ How small or big is your hurt? (Activities help the child to quantify the size of his hurt.)

➤ Does the hurt ever go away?

➤ When does it go away?

➤ Is there something you do that makes it go away?

➤ Is there something someone else does that makes it go away?

➤ Is there something or someone that makes the hurt come back?

➤ How long has that hurt been there?

➤ What happened that caused the hurt?

➤ Have you told anyone else about your hurt?

➤ What did they say to you about your hurt?

➤ If your hurt had a name, what name would you give it?

➤ If your hurt could talk, what do you think it would say to you?

➤ If it could listen, what would you say to it?

➤ Is there a song that would best describe what your hurt is like?

➤ Have you ever had a hurt like this before? If so, what happened?

➤ What would you like to see happen to the person or thing that caused the hurt?

➤ If you could do anything you wanted to that hurt, what would you do to it?

➤ What does your hurt look like? (A drawing activity helps the child portray his hurt, which then makes it easier for him to describe what that hurt is like.)

Answering any one of these questions, the child generally adds another reference for us to be curious about. If, for example, the child's response to our question, "If that hurt could talk, what would it say to you?" is "It would tell me it was my fault" our queries might be the following:

➤ What would make your hurt say that?

➤ What does your hurt think happened?

➤ What do you wish would have happened differently?

➤ What do you wish you would not have done at the time?

➤ What do you wish you might have done differently at the time?

➤ If your hurt could listen, what would you like to say back to it?

The Worst Part

The next subjective experience we present in the form of a question is, "What was the worst part?" This question often activates the old mindset and causes many to find it difficult to get started. They become stuck because they're thinking that they need to know the *worst part of what*, which is exactly what they ask the trainer. The reply to their question is, "You do not need to know *the what* in order to be curious. Just allow yourself

Point of Interest

A Broken Heart REALLY Feels Like It Is Breaking

A study (Kross, Berman, Mischel, Smith, & Wager, 2011) that compared 500 magnetic resonance imaging (MRI) scans of people's brain responses to physical pain, emotions, and other psychological processes reaffirms TLC's position that intense experiences of social rejection activate regions of the brain that are also involved in the sensory experience of physical pain. Basically, our brain interprets social rejection much like it interprets damage to the physical body.

Abandonment, neglect, verbal and emotional abuse, and bullying experiences are all extreme examples of rejection. Professionals often hear traumatized children complain about headaches, stomachaches, fatigue, and nausea; research findings help us to understand the connection. The experience of trauma is not a cognitive but rather a sensory experience. Our bodies have a memory, and while we may not readily be able to understand or make sense of why bad things happened, we do know that we hurt. Therefore, TLC trainings and interventions focus on exploring and delving into the themes of trauma that a child experiences, like fear or hurt.

TLC training provides immediately useable intervention strategies that encourage questions like, "Where in your body do you feel the hurt?" and "If the hurt was a color, what color would it be?" Validating that the hurt is real and concrete allows children to identify better ways to reduce and manage their hurt. For example, if a child indicates that her hurt lives in her chest and is the color blue, it becomes tangible. Once tangible, the child can learn how to be in control of the hurt, instead of the other way around. The goal is not to rid children of hurt forever, but to be able to regulate their feelings related to hurt when they surface.

to be curious about how the child experiences the worst part. After giving the groups a few minutes to list all of the questions they might ask, we again have each group give us just one of their questions and then keep returning until all of the questions are asked. Some of the questions include the following:

- ➣ Is the worst part still there?
- ➣ How small or big is the worst part?
- ➣ Have you ever had a worst part like this before?
- ➣ What happened that made this the worst part?
- ➣ Where were you when the worst part happened?
- ➣ What were you doing when the worst part happened?
- ➣ Were there others around when the worst part happened?
- ➣ What do you remember them doing?
- ➣ What reminds you of the worst part?

➤ Who reminds you of the worst part?

➤ What makes the worst part go away?

➤ What makes it come back?

➤ Who makes the worst part come back?

➤ Who helps make the worst part go away?

➤ What does the worst part make you want to do?

➤ Where do you feel the worst part the most in your body?

➤ Is there anything you do that makes it go away?

➤ Have you told anyone else about the worst part?

➤ What did they say to you when you told them?

➤ What do you wish you might have done differently when the worst part happened?

➤ What worries you the most about the worst part?

➤ What was the worst part of the worst part?

A response to any one of these questions could again lead to many more additional questions related to that part of the child's experience. If the child, for example, responds "I was watching" when asked what he was doing when the worst part happened, we would curiously pursue this with such questions as:

➤ What did you see?

➤ What stands out the most in your memory of what happened?

➤ What was the worst part of what you saw?

➤ What did it make you want to do?

➤ What did you do?

➤ What do you wish you could have done?

➤ How often do you still see what you saw in your mind?

Again, the child's response to any one of these questions could take us into an entirely different set of questions. The more curious we are, the more detail we learn about the child and what matters most.

Many more curious questions could be asked about the worst part without ever having any knowledge or case record histories of all that took place. When we put ourselves in the not knowing, curious role, we automatically move further into the child's world, rather than being in the distance because we are trying to make sense of the factual information or history we've gathered about that child.

If we return and review these lists of questions, we realize that we are giving children multiple opportunities to give their implicit memories a voice, to turn their sensations and feelings into something concrete that they can manage, talk to, and listen to, while we discover the meaning they have given their experiences, how these shape their view of themselves and others, and how they drive their behaviors. Once this is accomplished, children can more easily begin to reframe their experiences in ways that no longer terrify them but reflect their strength and resilience.

In reviewing this list, we also realize that several subjective experiences can be addressed simultaneously, as we do when we ask, "What worries you the most about your hurt?" This is similar to the child presenting us with two different references in response to one of our questions. In responding, for example, to the question of what reminds him of the worst part, the child might say, "It was when I saw my father and I heard the sirens." We would pursue both references by asking him to tell us more about

---

Magical Moment

One of the neatest moments was working with an 8-year old boy, who I will call Jay, whose father had committed suicide a year before. There was a lot of domestic violence in the home before this happened, and mom was actively using drugs. This boy was having severe behavior problems at school and was basically homeless after dad died. He went from house to house with mom, each situation not working for different reasons. Mom was jailed several times during that year, resulting in Jay staying with whoever would take him. Jay has two older sisters, one of whom mostly stayed where he did and the other who went and lived with other placements.

I saw Jay at his school. His favorite session was the Play-Doh activity, where he drew a picture of the person or thing that caused this horrible thing to happen. He placed the Play-Doh over the picture of the man he drew that he blamed for his dad's death, and pounded and pounded away. You could see the anger on his face as he put all of his energy into this activity. The next session we had moved on, but Jay asked if he could go back to that picture and use the Play-Doh again. He took his picture and put the Play-Doh on top of it again. He then proceeded to place the picture on the floor and began to stomp on it. He stomped and stomped until his fury was spent.

I continued to work with Jay and was able to complete the sessions with him. Near the end of our time together, we were working on the post-test to determine if he was experiencing some relief from his symptoms. He had scored very high on the scale of PTSD symptoms when we had begun. I was worried how it would turn out, because the school counselor had informed me that day that mom, Jay, and one of his sisters were in hiding because mom was running from the law again and had a warrant out for her arrest. Jay had missed several days of school while they tried to find him. As we were finishing up the post-test, I was noticing how much better his scores were and was amazed due to the constant chaos he lived in. I second-guessed myself in reply to one of his answers and said, "Are you sure?" His reply to me was, "Yep, I feel better now!" I smiled in amazement as I realized he had used the exact name of the program I was using to express his feelings, *I Feel Better Now!*

Jean West, LCSW, CTC-S, St. Joseph School District, Missouri

his father, and once he has no more to tell us about his father, we would then ask him to tell us more about those sirens; what he remembers about them, or when he hears sirens what they remind him of now, or what else happened when he heard the sirens.

When we present a third question to the group and tell them they ought to be able to identify 20 or 30 questions within a minute, it only takes a short time for the majority of the groups to realize the questioning process and many of its questions never really change; only the subjective experience we are curious about changes.

Summary

Being curious, allowing children to lead the process, and ensuring that they have multiple opportunities and the means to safely return to their subjective experiences in an empathetically, attuned, and in sync relationship are all part of the structured *SITCAP* process that helps us discover what matters most to children. As indicated several times, *SITCAP* is a structured process for the safety of children and their practitioners, but also to help ensure that children are not missing opportunities to bring us into their subjective worlds. Figures 5.6 and 5.7 reflect the value of this structured approach for practitioners working with traumatized children.

Figures 5.6 and 5.7   Before and after training

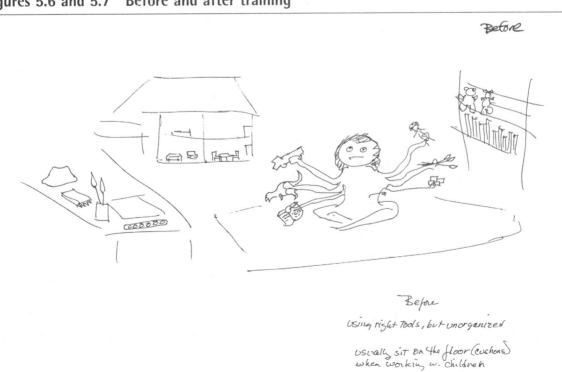

Before

Before
using right Tools, but unorganized

usually sit on the floor (cushions)
when working w. children

Figures 5.6 and 5.7   Continued

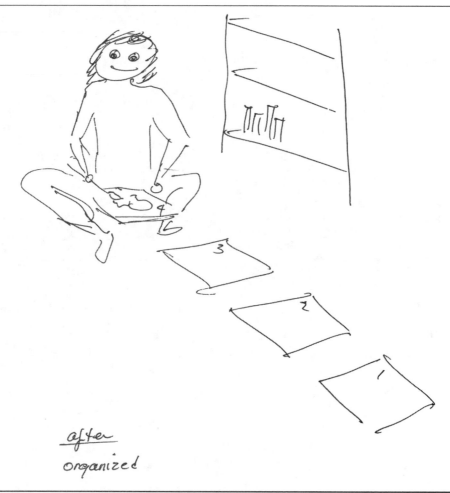

By maintaining a structured process, intervention fidelity is more easily maintained, and critical opportunities presented to traumatized children to define their subjective experiences and what matters most to them are not missed. We discover this in the next chapter as Emma, age 6; Peter, age 11; and Andrea, age 15, each take us into their worlds following the brutal murder of their sister. Following our journey with each of these children, we identify additional lessons learned. These three cases are also used to establish the four criteria needed to develop a solid strength-based and resilience-focused cognitive reframing of their experiences that they can accept and internalize.

CHAPTER Six

Meeting Children in Their World

In this chapter we present the stories of Emma, age 6; Peter, age 11; and Andrea, age 15. After each of their stories, we identify the key lessons learned emerging from our sessions with them. Their stories and the processes we detail further support the value of the *SITCAP* (*Structured Sensory Interventions for Traumatized Children, Adolescents and Parents*) process, not only for children but also for practitioners. We then use their stories to transition into our discussion about the use of cognitive reframing in the *SITCAP* process. Four reframing criteria are presented that are essential to constructing reframing statements that are meaningful and likely to be accepted and internalized by children. We introduce Sam, age 18, because his story illustrates the use of the fourth and most challenging, yet most influential, reframing criteria. We learn how the *SITCAP* reframing process is designed to help transform one's trauma from something that is feared to a resource of strength and hope.

In telling the stories of Emma, Peter, and Andrea, who were all from the same family, we use the pronoun "we" rather than "I" to reference the author's experiences when using *SITCAP* with these children. The worlds these children led us through are as alive today as they were years ago when we first met them. The lessons they taught us then remain an integral part of the *SITCAP* process today. Their drawings and stories reflect how children, who have been exposed to the violent experience and the loss of a loved one, reshape their view of themselves, each other, and how this new view impacts their behavior.

The Family: A Brutal Assault and Murder

Emma, Peter, and Andrea came to us one year following the brutal assault and murder of their 15-year-old sister, Elizabeth. Their single mother had limited support while trying to manage her own grief and trauma, as well as the impact this murder had on her children. For months following the murder, the media kept the story alive, making it difficult for the family to escape the constant reminders. In many ways, they experienced secondary trauma by the constant and prolonged replaying of details by the media.

All of the children developed their own unique reactions to their sister's murder and to the adjustments that now challenged them as a result of her absence. Prior to the murder, the family had been very close and supportive of one another. As we got to know them, it was clear that primary survival responses had shattered their previous closeness. Helping them find relief from the grief and terror of what they were experiencing was going to be necessary before they could reconnect with each other in supportive ways. Each of these children had brief counseling of a traditional nature that provided them support in the initial months that followed this brutal act, yet it did not prevent the primary reactions they were now displaying one year later.

Emma's Story

Emma was 5 years old when her sister was murdered. Developmentally, she did not understand what happened. She was not equipped to make sense of the long-term implications for her family. What she did experience was the abrupt disruption of the relationship she once enjoyed with her mother, sister, brother, and younger sister prior to the murder. Emma's mother reported that Emma had become very defiant, sassy, and was constantly fighting with her younger 4-year-old sister. Because we focus on the experience, rather than symptoms, and have learned over the years that this intervention reveals reactions that are not always observable, it was not necessary to assign her reactions to either grief or trauma for the intervention to be helpful. What mattered the most was to give Emma a vehicle and a medium that would allow her to reveal what mattered most to her. Initially, she was given the option to tell us what happened and how things changed for her at home or to draw. She decided, with no hesitation, to draw.

When Emma was asked to draw a picture of what happened that she could tell us a story about, she actually drew a picture of her face but not the rest of her body. This is where our curiosity began. We asked her what she liked, the things she did not like, and then what she remembered most about her sister. When asked what she missed most about her sister, she simply said, "The games she played with me." After asking questions related to her drawing, we then asked, "Where's the rest of you?" She replied, "Nowhere." There could have been a variety of responses that provided us with more of an understanding of how she was experiencing her sister's absence, but in this case Emma responded very literally to our question. She was then asked if she could draw the rest of her body, which she did. It was fully intact with hands and feet. While she drew, she talked about her favorite things to do and eat.

Emma's next task was to draw a picture of how she imagined her sister looked dead. Again she only drew her sister's face, and again our curiosity pursued what else she could tell us about her sister. When asked about the rest of her sister's body, she said nothing but picked up the colored pencils and began drawing the rest of her body. In the process of drawing her, she said, "I'm going to color her just like me." Emma's mother explained to us that the she was quite close with Elizabeth and that the two really enjoyed being together.

We will be learning more about Emma, but as is common in this process, we were not quite sure when Emma might take us deeper into her world until she was asked to draw a picture of her family doing something. Asking children to draw a picture of their family doing something is much safer for them than asking them to just draw a picture of the family. Many traumatized families have secrets that are taboo. Drawing the family doing something (Figure 6.1) allows the child to focus on the activity, thereby taking the focus off whatever emotional issues, secrets, and taboos might exist in the family. It was this drawing and the story Emma told about her family that revealed what mattered most to her.

Emma's drawing represents her mother on the left side of the page, her brother Peter in the middle, and her sister Andrea on the right side of the page. Emma described what the family was doing but left herself out of the activity and the drawing, so she was asked, "Where are you?" At this point she took her finger and put it on the drawing of her mother in the area of her mother's stomach and then simply said, "I'm here." In our trainings we ask participants what they would ask Emma at this point. Those still struggling with allowing themselves to be curious cannot answer, whereas those who are able to be curious simply follow the child's lead and reply, "Where is here?" She responded immediately, "I'm inside my mommy's tummy." Somewhat surprised by her response, we said, "Wow, that's interesting" and then paused for a moment because it was a bit hard to stop the old mindset from wondering what this was all about instead of simply following her lead. We then asked her, "What's it like in your mommy's tummy?" Emma replied with a very big smile and a good deal of animation, "I'm the only one there. There is no one else. Wherever mommy goes, I go."

Figure 6.1   The family doing something

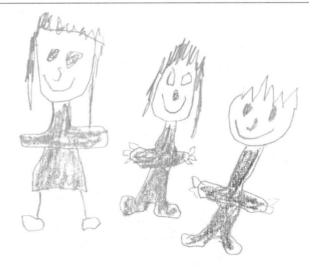

In this curious journey, Emma, who has been defiant, oppositional, sassy, and fighting with her younger sister, tells us how good she feels being with her mother; not only being with her mother but having her mother's attention, comfort, and protection. Although we are not yet finished with this intervention, this one drawing provided us with a window into Emma's world and revealed what she needed most. Her mother, who was observing the interview behind a one-way mirror, as it was also being video-taped for training, said to the trauma specialist spending time with her, "Oh my god, she wants more of my attention; that's what this is all about" (meaning her behavior). When parents or guardians actually hear how their children are experiencing what happened, they frequently understand what they need to do differently in order to make a difference in how their children behave.

We continued to talk about what it was like for Emma to be in her mommy's tummy until she had no more to say. If you recall the house fire example in Chapter 5, we stated that if the child places us outside of an event we need to go inside, or if placed inside that environment, in this case mommy's tummy, we need to eventually move the story to the outside environment. At one point, Emma said she was kicking, so we asked, "Are you kicking to get out?" but she said she was not. She talked a bit more about her favorite things to do with her mother, and then we asked if she could draw a picture of herself outside of mommy's tummy. Emma asked if we wanted her to draw herself as a baby. We replied, "You can draw yourself however you like." She drew herself as a baby and continued to talk about how nice it was to be that baby. Shortly afterward, she abruptly put her pencil down on the table and simply said, "I'm done."

The interview was concluded a few minutes later after she was thanked for being so helpful and asked if there was anything else she would like to tell us. She had no more to tell. When she was reunited with her mother, they engaged in a long hug that both had needed for some time. Her mother now knew what was important to Emma and, in the months that followed, she and her mother began enjoying what they had enjoyed before the murder. Emma's presenting behaviors all but disappeared, except when mom needed a reminder or Emma needed a little more attention.

Lessons Learned

➤ We never know which drawing activity will take us to the center of the child's world, or when. In this case, it was not Emma's self-portrait or the drawing of her sister Elizabeth, but the drawing of her family doing something that brought us into her world.

➤ By being curious and following Emma into her world, in this case mommy's tummy, we discover what matters most to her. When bringing Emma outside of her mommy's tummy, she draws herself as a baby and in her own way emphasizes to us how important it is for her to re-experience the attention, care, and connection she had with her mother before it was abruptly ended by her sister's murder.

➤ If mother had not also been a witness to her daughter's inner world, our recommendations that she needed to spend more time with her daughter would likely be dismissed, minimized, or met with responses like, "Yes, but how will this change anything? Are you saying it was my fault?" Being a witness makes it much easier to understand and accept what matters most.

➤ Drawing provided Emma a vehicle to communicate what she could not verbalize.

➤ Whether her reactions were grief or trauma driven did not matter; what mattered was making us a witness to what she needed to experience to be happy again.

➤ No amount of verbal interaction would have altered Emma's behavior.

Peter's Story

Peter's primary reaction was much different than that of his younger sister. At age 11, like many children exposed to violence, he had become hypervigilant and activated by various environmental factors that reminded him of what happened. Most troublesome for Peter's mother and for Peter was his aggressive behavior and fighting. Mom reported that, prior to the murder, Peter got along with everyone, had many friends, and loved to laugh. One year after the murder, the laughter was gone, many of his previous friends were no longer friends, and he was getting into fights. It is important to keep in mind that Peter is the only male in his family. As his experience unfolds, this will have meaning related to his behavior.

Peter was asked if he would like to tell us a bit of what happened before starting his drawings. He agreed and easily began sharing the details of what happened. He began telling us about the last few minutes he spent with his sister before she was assaulted and killed. Peter responded quite freely to our curiosity about what he knew. Halfway into this initial 15-minute discussion, the free-flowing manner in which he was giving information stopped. He began having a stuttering-like response, finding it difficult to form the words that detailed what he knew about his sister being stabbed to death multiple times. When the words came, so did the tears. His pain and underlying fear, even one year later, were still quite observable. When the tears subsided, his reactions were briefly normalized, and then he was given the choice to stop at this point or do some drawing for us. He decided to draw. His first drawing was used in Chapter 4 (Figure 4.6) to compare with his younger sister's drawing to illustrate that it doesn't matter what a child draws; every line and every scribble contains elements of the child's experience. He used this first drawing to tell us more of what he remembered before his sister left for the park "never to come back."

Figure 6.2, his second drawing, contains several different drawings because he insisted on using the same sheet of paper to complete two different tasks, even though

Figure 6.2   Peter before and after the murder

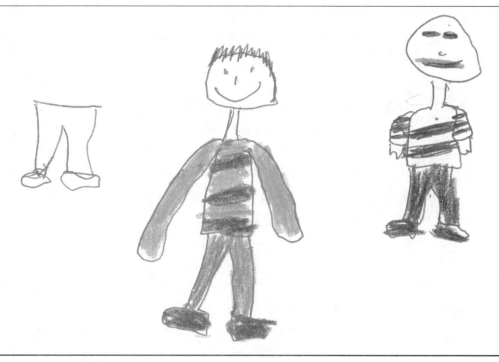

he was offered additional paper. The first picture he draws is of himself in the upper-right corner of the paper. When asked if this was a picture of him before or after the murder, he indicated it was a picture of him before the murder. He described some of the things he liked to do before all this happened and some of the things he remembered doing with his sister. Because this was a picture of Peter *before* the murder, we offered him another sheet of paper to draw a picture of himself *now*. He said he would use the same sheet of paper and drew the lower part of his body on the left side of the paper, but then he abruptly stopped and said, "I don't like the way I'm drawing this." Again he was offered another sheet of paper, but again he refused. (When children are given the "container" [paper] in which to put their trauma, they are empowered by determining what they will or will not put into it. It is not unusual for them to use the same sheet of paper to start over when their first attempt is not what they like. However, some will ask for more paper until they get their drawing the way they want.)

The self-portrait in the center of the paper is of Peter one year after the murder. When presented in training, practitioners immediately cite how powerful his arms look and the difference between how his face looks in the drawing of himself *then* and *now*. We caution here that it is important not to interpret what they see, that the only validity of what they are looking at is what the child tells us his drawing represents. Peter indicated that he still thinks about what happened to his sister and that it sometimes wakes him up at night. When asked about the face he drew, he indicated, "I just drew it that way because I should be smiling." He had no more to tell at this point, so he was asked if he could draw a picture of what happened.

Figure 6.3, the stick figure closest to the car, represents his sister, who was being stabbed to death by her killer. Because of the lengthy media coverage of this case, the amount of detail Peter provided about what happened was not surprising. What was surprising, however, is where this drawing took us. One of the trauma-specific experiences we pursue is the fear and/or the terror experienced at the time of the trauma and how it is being experienced even months, or in this case one year, later. After describing what scared him the most *then*, he was asked what scared him the most *now*. At this point, he took us into an entirely different experience. He started this new experience with, "I was in court when they brought him [the killer] in the court." This now became a story within a story but did much to explain and support his hypervigilance, increasing aggressiveness, and fighting.

Being curious, we explored what he remembered the most about that day in court, who else was there, and what happened. He was asked if he could draw a picture of his sister's killer, but he said he could not. He went into a great deal of detail about coming face to face with his sister's killer, but he never answered the question of what scares him the most *now*. When we restated our question about what scares him the most *now* since this happened, then his behavior and portrayal of himself *now* makes sense. He replied, "That [the killer] would break out of jail and come kill the rest of my family."

When trainees hear this part of the story, they immediately return to his previous drawing of himself with those big, powerful arms, mention his hypervigilant, aggressive behavior, and realize that, in his world, the only way Peter can feel safe is to feel powerful. The role of the male as being the protector also influences this position. Intervention therefore needed to engage Peter in experiences that allowed him to feel empowered in

Figure 6.3   What happened

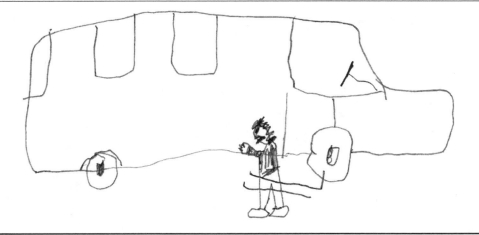

ways that were not self-defeating and that helped him learn to regulate his fear. The *SITCAP* process is designed to help children accomplish this task.

In his final drawing, Figure 6.4, he drew a picture of what his sister looked like dead at the bottom of the page. He provided additional details about what happened to her body. One of his responses caused us to ask him to draw a picture of what she looked like before her death. The face at the top of the page is a picture of her before the murder. He talked about some of the fun things he remembered about her. *SITCAP* is designed so we move in and out of the trauma memories to fond memories, fun activities, or *safe places* as a way to titrate the focus on trauma. Often times, like Peter, children will do this for us. There is one additional common, subjective experience we give Peter the opportunity to address. Because he did not initiate any reference to the hurt he may have experienced when all this happened, we asked, "When this first happened or when you first found out, where did you feel the hurt the most in your body?" He responded immediately, "in my head." He indicated that he had severe headaches for some time after the murder, but now he only gets these headaches when he is "out in the sun too long." When asked, "So when you think of your sister now, where do you feel the hurt the most?" he replied that he felt it mostly in his stomach.

When asked if he could describe what that hurt was like, he attempted to do so using some examples from horror movies. When he no longer had anything else to tell us about his hurt, we spent the last 15 minutes of the session having him describe what he liked

Figure 6.4   What the hurt looks like

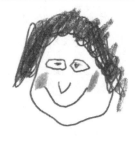

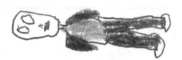

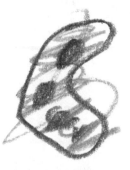

doing the most now. We laughed a bit and let him know several things he could do to help himself. We indicated that if there was no one he felt comfortable talking with, the one thing he could do that might help when he was having a hard time was to do what we did today—draw. To our surprise, he immediately began drawing the figure in the lower-right corner of Figure 6.4. When he was finished, he said without hesitation, "You know that hurt we were talking about, this is what the hurt looks like. It's like your guts being ripped out. It feels like someone is eating you."

Earlier we had asked him only to describe his hurt, not to externalize it and put it into a concrete form. This is a wonderful example of how Peter *reciprocated* by teaching us how this is such an important part of the healing process. In essence, he was saying he needed for us to see what his hurt was like in order to feel better. Drawing what the hurt might look like is a standard activity in *SITCAP*. How children depict their hurt and other reactions can vary significantly, as well as be depicted in very similar ways. However, what is most important is the meaning children give to what they draw.

The intensity at the beginning of the interview, when Peter was still living with the pain and terror of what happened, had diminished significantly. The turning point of our understanding of what his life was like was certainly answered in his responses to what scared him the most *now*. From that point on, he no longer struggled with his words, but he was talking freely and laughing. Weeks later, his mother reported that Peter was beginning to be much more like himself. We consulted with his social worker, encouraging a focus on involving Peter in activities that would give him a sense of empowerment. In the months that followed, his earlier survival behaviors all but diminished.

Lessons Learned

> Attempting to process traumatic events by direct verbal intervention alone can at times intensify the reactions because they remain internalized, intangible, and unmanageable, rather than outside ourselves in a concrete manageable form.

> An 8-by-11 piece of paper empowers a child to take control of how to best externalize and manage his traumatic memories. Peter insisted on using the same sheet of paper for his drawing.

> By allowing Peter to lead us into his world, his behavior makes sense as we discover, by being curious and following his story into the courtroom, that he is living in constant fear.

> Peter was not only living in terror but also experiencing a good deal of hurt that would not have emerged had we not asked trauma-specific questions about his hurt. This is why we integrate into each *SITCAP* session a focus on one of the subjective experiences of trauma.

> Peter dramatically illustrates how helpful it is to not just talk, in this case about the hurt, but to be able to externalize that subjective experience into a concrete form that

can be given a context in which to more easily communicate what that experience is like and get relief from it.

➤ The more we learn about a child's subjective experience, the easier it becomes to construct relevant reframing statements. (This will be discussed in the upcoming section on cognitive reframing.)

Andrea's Story

When we met with Andrea she was 15, the same age as her sister was when she was murdered. They were the best of friends, shared a bedroom, and traveled in the same circle of friends. This was a sudden and traumatic loss for everyone, but especially for Andrea. Emotionally, she shut down immediately, became detached and numb. This was such a painful and horrible loss for her that she needed to avoid all reminders. Just being alone in the bedroom she and her sister had shared was often too painful for Andrea. Shortly after the funeral, Andrea removed everything from the bedroom that reminded her of her sister and no longer associated with past friends. Neither her mother nor other family members understood the avoidant behaviors Andrea engaged in, which left Andrea with very little support. In some ways, Andrea's mother looked to her daughter for help and comfort, both of which Andrea found difficult to give. At times Andrea would not come home. She would call her mother to say she was okay but not coming home. This event, combined with such a challenging developmental period in her life, was becoming quite overwhelming for Andrea.

Andrea did not hesitate to draw. In the first few activities she was also responsive to our questions regarding details of the murder, but she had difficulty when asked questions about what it was like for her. Andrea had a wonderful smile and was engaging very early in the session. Later, we learned that every time someone asked her how she was doing it would reactivate her pain, so she quickly learned to put people off with her smile and engaging manner. Her avoidant behaviors told a much different story. At one point, after drawing a picture of herself, she was asked, "When you look at yourself now, what do you see?" Her response was, "I need to fix my hair." At least halfway into the session, her reply to our curiosity reflected a similar *disconnect* from her inner world. When asked the future orientation question, "When you think about it, what do you see yourself doing in the future?" she could not respond. There was no verbal response. After a brief silence, we reflected, "That made you stop and think for a moment." She had nothing to say. Andrea could not afford to think about the future, only the moment in time in which she was living. Going back to when she and her sister shared so much was far too painful, and thoughts about the future stopped the day her sister, her very best friend, was murdered.

Never knowing where in this process or what activity or focus will become helpful to the child, we simply presented one activity after another. We let her lead us to what she could communicate, and when there was no more to tell us, we moved on. The turning point came when we asked her to draw a picture of her sister dead (Figure 6.5). At first she said she didn't know how to draw her sister. We reminded her that it did not matter what she drew or how she drew. She sat quietly for a moment and then said, "I don't know what to draw about her. I could describe what she looked like better." Remembering how helpful it was for Peter to make us a witness to what his hurt was like, we wanted Andrea to try to externalize her memories. However, we have also learned from children over the years that there can be many symbolic, implicit memories, making it difficult to select one memory to begin with; at times we just need to give children a starting point. We suggested to Andrea that she might just want to start with her sister's face and go from there. The moment we gave Andrea a singular focus, she immediately began drawing but started by drawing the car. When she finished drawing the car, she drew her sister, the stick figure closest to the car. The other stick figure represents her killer.

Andrea went on to provide details about what she knew happened. It was actually easier for her to give us details about what happened versus what this experience was like for her. At about 30 minutes into this 60-minute session, Andrea indicated that her mother would not allow her to go to the morgue to see her sister one last time when her body was being identified. Andrea was upset with her mother, but more importantly was left with her own image of what her stepsister must have looked like. Andrea had maintained fairly consistent eye contact up to this point. However, when asked to tell us a little bit more about her sister, she lowered her head and kept her gaze on her drawing. This again was a very simplistic stick figure but one filled with memories. Tears began to roll down her face as we sat there silently. When asked what she was remembering, she responded, "We used to do everything together. We used to race, but she always won

Figure 6.5   Deceased sister

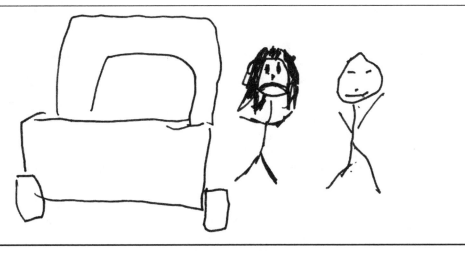

because she was faster than me. We always had so much fun together." Andrea continued crying and verbalizing the times they had shared together. She was no longer detached, no longer avoiding the deep sadness resulting from that part of her life that was so horribly and abruptly ended. Both Andrea and her mother reported that these were the very first tears Andrea had shed since the murder. The release of this sadness one year later brought her some relief. It was a new beginning for her.

Lessons Learned

➤ Children can have so many implicit memories that, when asked to begin to externalize them through drawing, it may be difficult for them to know where to begin. Often all they need to start drawing is for us to give them a specific focus point.

➤ When implicit memories are externalized into a concrete form, even as a nondescriptive stick figure, children can more safely and easily express what they could not previously express or put into words.

➤ Putting symbolic memories into a concrete form can help reattach victims to those feelings and memories that were too painful or overwhelming to allow themselves to have at the time of what happened.

Although these examples were only one session in length, they illustrate *SITCAP*'s core processes. These processes remain the same for even the more difficult cases, which we described in the earlier chapters using evidence-based research to document the gains those children also made using this process.

Following Intervention

This family had become fragmented and disconnected after the murder. All of these children were struggling in their own way to just survive. Their behavior was driven by the pain and terror this brutal murder had caused. As the mother witnessed how each of her children are now experiencing their lives, she realized that their behaviors were being driven by their individual experiences. It allowed her to become more nurturing, protective, and much less reactive. She understood now that trying to control their behavior by punishment only made it worse for her children and for herself. She learned that their behaviors were in response to feeling needed, comforted, and empowered, which she was now empowered to provide. As a result, the family began reconnecting with each other and working together to make a new life for themselves. Andrea and Peter's troubling behaviors all but disappeared with additional brief, trauma-focused intervention. Emma responded immediately to her mother's efforts and did not need additional help.

Cognitive Reframing

In *SITCAP*, reframing is not initiated until the end of the session. The primary reason for this is that until we spend time in the child's world, we cannot possibly know what may be a meaningful reframing that fits the context in which the child is experiencing himself and his environment—a reframing that empowers the child to think and behave differently.

Reframing can address subjective experiences in a generalized way. Following is a generalized reframing for worry: "Everyone worries at times, but worries come and go like a storm. Like a storm, worries at times can be very worrisome, but then like a storm they too pass. The storm comes, stays awhile, and then it stops and the sun comes out. When our worries are really big, we can remember that, like a storm, the best thing that we can do while worrying is to make sure we are safe and then keep ourselves busy doing something until the storm or our worries pass." This general statement is to be followed by identifying what the child could do while waiting for his worries to go away. In *SITCAP* there are several different reframing statements for worry that speak to varied aspects of worry and lead into different activities to support the reframing. There are generalized reframing statements for each of the subjective experiences included in the intervention. For some children, this generalized reframing will be helpful. However, it is only the beginning of our reframing efforts.

For traumatized children, the pain, hurt, fear, and worries can be so intense and constant that our efforts to help them reframe the way they think about themselves in order to help them ultimately begin regulating their reactions must be personalized. For reframing statements to be personal and more likely to be accepted as making sense and thereafter internalized by the child, they must include one or more of the following four criteria:

1. Matches the child's developmental level of understanding
2. Directly references how the child is subjectively experiencing what is happening or happened
3. Matches the conclusions the child may have arrived at following *SITCAP*'s structured sensory activities
4. Presented in a way that transforms the trauma from something that is feared to a resource that empowers the child to see self, others, and life through a lens of hope, strength, and resilience

The more of these criteria that are included in the reframing, the stronger that reframing will be, and the more likely it is to be accepted by the child and integrated into how the child thinks about himself and ultimately how he begins to behave.

Developmentally Appropriate Reframing

An example of a reframing that matches the child's developmental level of understanding is the reframing given to Emma. Attempting to reframe for Emma the meaning of her behavior as a survival response or a behavior she uses to get her mother to respond differently is accurate, but not one a 6-year-old is likely to appreciate or grasp in a way that would change the way she was thinking and behaving. Presenting Emma the following reframing is more likely to be accepted, as it was by Emma: "Emma, when you were talking about how nice it was to be in your mommy's tummy, you were really happy. You really liked it. You know whenever you're sad, mad, or even scared, you can go back to your mommy's tummy like you did today and remember what it was like, and that will help you feel better. You can even say to your mother, 'Mommy, I want to feel like a baby,' and she will then know what she needs to do to help you feel better." This is a reframing Emma understood, because it was presented in age-appropriate language and also because it was a "place" where she spent remembering, one that was emotionally pleasurable.

Directly Referencing the Experience

We use Peter as an example of how we can directly reference the child's subjective experience to make that reframing statement more meaningful. If Peter had not directly made us a witness to what his hurt was like, we would have no reference on which to construct a personalized reframing that spoke directly to his subjective experience of hurt. If that were actually the case, we would need to use a more generalized reframing in the hopes that it would be meaningful to him. However, Peter's reference to his hurt did allow us to arrive at a personal and meaningful reframing using the context that he used to describe his hurt. He said his hurt was, "Like having your guts ripped out; that's what it feels like."

The reframing we constructed was, "You know, Peter, when something or someone causes you to feel the way you described your hurt, think of it as your body's way of saying that whatever has been happening in your life has really been so hard that it's time to let someone know what has been happening. If there is no one you feel comfortable talking to at the time, you can also draw what it's like for you, like we did today, so you can feel better and get some relief from it, like you also did today." This is a reframing he accepted, because it matched his subjective experience. It is also one that empowers him to do something to regulate his body's reaction to what has been or is happening. Helpful reframing statements will include several of the four criteria cited, as just seen in both Emma's and Peter's examples.

A Conclusion Already Reached

We use Andrea's situation to demonstrate that when a reframing statement reflects the conclusion the child has already reached following the sensory activity just completed, it is more likely to be accepted and internalized and to positively influence the way the child feels, thinks, and later behaves. As Andrea was able to return to the good times she and her sister shared, her body was able to begin to relieve itself of the sadness that had been frozen deep inside her painful world for the past year. At the same time,

Andrea later indicated that it felt good to return to those memories. Reframing this conclusion, we simply used her experience to help her think about herself and her life differently. What made sense to her was, "Andrea, as you replayed the good times the two of you had together, it brought tears, because your time together was abruptly ended. At the same time, it felt good to remember what you both enjoyed so much. Those memories really are to be enjoyed and treasured for a lifetime, not avoided or forgotten." This was a reframing Andrea easily accepted, because she had arrived at that conclusion for herself. This was an empowering reframing, because we also addressed her avoidant behavior when we added that the memories were "not to be avoided but enjoyed." It also provided a foundation for us in subsequent sessions to transition to her beginning to build new, treasured memories with others.

Transforming the Trauma: Sam's Story

The example we use to illustrate the importance of constructing a reframing that transforms that child's trauma from something that is feared to a resource that empowers is the story of Sam. It should be noted that this fourth criteria is one of the most difficult to construct. As we tell Sam's story, we realize that the quality and value of what we reframe is also based on what we know or do not know about that child's view of his future.

Sam was 18 years old. He was a high school senior who was severely beaten while ushering at a large movie complex theater. In the weeks that followed his beating, he isolated himself and withdrew from his friends, school, and the activities he once enjoyed. He was a muscular teen who was on the first string of his school's football team. He was due to graduate in the early spring and had been accepted into the police academy. The beating he experienced now threatened his future and, in many ways, his own life. Sam was very active in his church youth group until the beating. He had withdrawn from those activities as well, and shortly after the attack he had told his parish priest he was going to give up going to the police academy. The parish priest's efforts to reason with him failed. Approximately six weeks after the attack, the priest called us for help.

Sam agreed, somewhat reluctantly, to meet with us through the encouragement of the parish priest but mostly his football coach. The intervention process was explained to him. His reactions were normalized, and he was given the options to say *yes* or *no* to responding to whatever we might ask him about or activities we might ask him to complete. Sam began by telling us a little bit about what happened.

He was ushering at the large movie complex on New Year's Eve. There were 15 different movies playing. Each of the small theaters in the complex was completely filled. Sam had made several attempts to get control of three teens disturbing those around them. He had little success. At one point he asked his manager for help, but the manager indicated that he was way too busy and that Sam would have to manage on his own. When the movie in the theater he was responsible for ended, so did several of the other movies in his area. People began exiting from a half-dozen of the theaters in his part of the complex. When the three teens Sam had unsuccessfully confronted saw him outside the door of their theater, they immediately rushed him, knocked him to the ground, and began kicking and stomping on him. Getting his head stomped into a marble floor could have caused significant brain damage. He was fortunate in this regard but was hospitalized with multiple fractures, abrasions, and a concussion. The beating happened suddenly. There was no shouting back and forth, just the immediate attack. His physical wounds were healing, but the sensory memories and emotions of this sudden attack remained intense.

Sam drew what happened and gave some details about the physical aspects of his experience. When he was finished, he was asked, "What was the worst part of what happened?" When we present this example in training, several possibilities are mentioned by attendees, including the manager not helping, the attack happening so quickly that Sam couldn't defend himself, that Sam's view of himself as smart and tough was shattered, that perhaps he experienced a great deal of shame, that he was subjected to ridicule at school by those who did not like him, that he was blamed for what happened by people wondering out loud how he could let this happen, the physical pain he experienced, and the thoughts that he might die or be permanently injured.

Sam's response was quite different, demonstrating again that we may think we know what a child experienced, but often we do not. In response to our question about the worst part, Sam said, "I'm on the floor. They're kicking and stomping on me. As they are kicking and stomping on me, I can see between their legs and as I look between their legs, I see all these people standing around and no one is helping me." Although Sam's beating took less than two minutes before the teens ran off, the experience was still very much alive. He experienced an overwhelming sense of powerlessness and fear for his life. Equally as devastating was the lack of response from the adults watching. His withdrawal and isolation were certainly understandable from his perspective, but was also worrisome because of his indication earlier that he was not going to enroll in the police academy.

Near the end of the interview, Sam was asked about his not wanting to attend the police academy. His response was, "If I can't take care of myself, how can I take care of anyone else?" So not only was he giving up on others, but he was also giving up on himself and his future. This raised concern about suicide, which he did deny having, but it certainly might be a realization if his isolation, withdrawal, and his powerless, helpless view of himself continued.

Point of Interest

Reframing Children's Behaviors

When children's behaviors are challenging, it is helpful to understand how the parent may see it and then provide the parent with an alternate way to view the behavior. This is often the first step in helping parents respond to behaviors in ways that are more strength-based and trauma-informed.

WHINING:

➤ A parent may see the behavior as, "She is doing it to get my attention. She is being manipulative."

➤ Another way to frame this behavior is to say, "She is trying to practice expressing her needs. She is showing great control over frustrations and a lack of words to tell you what is really making her upset."

SAYING "NO" AND TESTING LIMITS:

➤ A parent may see the behavior as, "She is so oppositional and defiant."

➤ Another way to frame this behavior is to say, "She is becoming an independent person. She is trying to tell you that she has a mind of her own."

NEGATIVE BEHAVIORS LIKE PUSHING, HITTING, BITING:

➤ A parent may see the behavior as, "She thinks if she throws a fit she will get her way. She is mean."

➤ Another way to frame this behavior is to say, "She is telling you that she has lost control and needs your help."

DISPLAYING NEW FEARS:

➤ A parent may see the behavior as, "She is always afraid of something; I can't take her anywhere."

➤ Another way to reframe this behavior is to say, "She is starting to think about lots of new things, and sometimes that gets scary."

Reframing the Experience

The urgency of trying to reframe Sam's experience as a resource that would enhance his future as a police officer was now essential. However, constructing any reframing statement that was personally specific to his experience and directed at reconnecting him to the future would likely fail or fall short if aspects of his being a cop could not be integrated into that reframing. I have a son who is a police officer, and this provided the reference needed to construct a reframing that would help Sam use his experience as a resource. It can honestly be said that had it not been for my own experiences with police officers, the following reframing simply would not have been constructed. The reality is that there will always be numerous times when our efforts to reframe are limited by our own knowledge and experience and require that we consult with colleagues who are familiar with the different aspects of that child's experience.

I, Dr. Steele, knew Sam had accompanied several police officers on their shifts while on patrol. I began the reframing by asking him a question that again would not have been available to me without my own experiences with police procedures. I asked Sam, "I know you've been on patrol rides and obviously know your protocols since you were accepted into the academy. I wonder if you could tell me why it is standard protocol to call and wait for backup to arrive before entering into a dangerous situation?" He thought for a moment and then replied, "I guess because anyone can be taken out." Had he not given this response, I would have framed it for him in hopes of being able to move him from being stuck with his subjective view of himself as helpless and incapable of taking care of anyone, to one who would make a good cop and an excellent partner. His response told me he was going to be okay, but it certainly needed to be expanded in a way that it would become personally meaningful and supported by his desire to become a cop. The reframing I constructed was, "You are absolutely right. It doesn't matter how tough you are, how big you are, how smart you are; the one valuable lesson you have painfully learned is that there is safety in numbers. And the one thing I know with absolute certainty is that you're going to make one heck of a cop and one heck of a partner because you now really understand this."

This was a turning point for Sam. His experience now became a resource, a reason why he would make a good cop. It reconnected him to his future and now gave a purpose to his experience. Had I not had that information or that reference as a result of my experiences via my son the cop, my efforts to construct such a personal, empowering reframing simply would not have happened.

We strongly encourage practitioners to construct reframing statements by incorporating as many of the four criteria listed as possible. This is not always easy, as Sam's story illustrated. However, integration of even one or two of these criteria makes for a much more meaningful reframing and one that is more likely to be internalized by the child. The *SITCAP* process is designed to reveal the kinds of references and descriptions of subjective experiences that can be used to enhance the quality and value of our reframing efforts.

Magical Moment

Most recently, I was working with an elementary student with severe behavior problems. I met with her twice, and the changes in her behavior were almost instant, especially with her extreme and excessive stealing behaviors. Interestingly, her mother was incarcerated for stealing. After two sessions, the student was no longer stealing. Following our second session, her teacher and our staff asked me, "What have you done with this student? She is like a different child." *SITCAP* really works! I have seen nothing less than amazing results using the *SITCAP* interventions.

Mary Langstrand, MSW, PLCSW, CTS; School Social Worker,
Wake County Public School System, Cary, North Carolina

Summary

The essential process and components of *SITCAP* have now been addressed in detail. The programs are so structured that each session can be easily implemented. The process itself is not difficult, but it requires a *mind shift* that is best accomplished with brief practice, as we demonstrated in the previous chapter. *SITCAP*'s healing value is substantially supported by evidence-based research and practice history in varied settings with children presenting with varied violent and nonviolent, yet trauma-inducing, situations. As illustrated, *SITCAP* integrates both sensory and cognitive processes that support what we know about the neuroscience of trauma today. In the next chapter, we examine *SITCAP*'s use in schools, where children are the most accessible for intervention and where school-related incidents can induce trauma.

CHAPTER Seven

Incorporating *SITCAP* in Schools and Community-Based Organizations

In this chapter we review the recovery protocols and interventions that TLC developed, recommends, and uses following a school's response to a traumatic incident. TLC's recovery protocols and interventions are implemented in order to prevent the development of PTSD in students and staff or, when needed, are made available to those experiencing trauma reactions and symptoms despite earlier intervention efforts. They are designed to also prevent inappropriate interventions and responses resulting from misinterpreting the meaning of behaviors of those in crisis and, as discussed in this chapter, they are necessary to help prevent the need for trauma-specific intervention in the future. However, these interventions are also necessary to best determine which students in the weeks that follow these earlier interventions may benefit from *SITCAP* (*Structured Sensory Interventions for Traumatized Children, Adolescents and Parents*).

Although our discussion is specific to schools, we use the same processes when asked to assist community-based children's programs and youth organizations that have experienced a traumatic incident. Before introducing our recommended interventions, it is important to present a more detailed description of the impact trauma has on learning and behavior than that presented in Chapter 3, in order to best support the provision of these timely and appropriate trauma-informed interventions in school settings.

Trauma's Impact on Learning

Millions of school-age children and adolescents enter school every day already traumatized. In addition, thousands more are exposed to trauma through school-related incidents such as violence, bullying, suicide, and the sudden accidental death of students or staff. At least 14% of all children, and more than 65% in some environments, are exposed to trauma; of those who are exposed, an estimated 36% develop PTSD (Alisic, van der Schoot, van Ginkel, & Kleber, 2008; APA, 2000; Copeland, Anglod, & Costello, 2007; Fletcher, 2003). If our primary objective in schools is to help children learn, then we must understand how trauma impacts learning and behavior in order to better afford traumatized students those interventions that can help restore their learning capacity.

As early as 1992, it was reported that trauma negatively impacts short-term memory (Starkman, Gebarski, Berent, & Schteingart, 1992). Bremner, Krystal, Charnez, and Southwick (1996) reported that abused children had lower memory volumes than did nontraumatized children. Perry and Szalavitz (2006) and others indicated that traumatized children have difficulty with processing verbal information, attending, focusing, retaining, and recalling information (Bremner, 2001; Saigh & Bremner, 1999; Starkman et al., 1992). Cognitive deficits such as poor problem solving (unable to think things out or make sense of what is happening), low self-esteem (how one thinks about himself), hopelessness (loss of future orientation), and powerlessness (the inability to take action to help one's self) are all clearly linked to negative, traumatic life events (LeDoux, 2002; Nader, 2008; Schore, 2001; Stien & Kendall, 2004; Teicher, 2000).

When children are in trauma, they experience their world *implicitly* from the limbic midbrain areas of the brain. Reason, logic, and the abilities to understand, process, and learn are difficult to access when in trauma, as these are *explicit* neocortex functions (Fishbane, 2007). As a result of these trauma-influenced changes, children develop a rigid cognitive style that conflicts with their efforts to learn (Ford, Chapman, Mack, & Pearson, 2006).

When children are functioning from the limbic region, their intense fear also triggers the primary survival behaviors of fight, flight, and freeze. These survival behaviors, generated by untreated trauma, directly complicate learning and further compromise students' abilities to focus and stay on task. Traumatized students are not able to communicate their fears with words, but they do so through behavioral outbursts and disruptive behaviors. Unfortunately, such behaviors can be misinterpreted as being disrespectful and defiant, or as ADHD, mood disorders, and many other diagnoses that are often erroneously assigned to traumatized children.

Trauma's Impact on Behavior

Traumatized students respond quickly to teachers or school personnel who are beginning to lose control, indicated by a change in breathing pattern, facial expression, or tonal voice changes (Brendtro et al., 2009). These cues trigger perceptions of pending threat for traumatized students and activate their primitive, instinctive survival responses. Such midbrain survival reactions by students are not rational or by choice, as they are not generated by the neocortex or thinking, rational brain; instead, they are sensory reactions generated by the nonthinking limbic system. One student's alarm reaction can also trigger and spread to other students, creating a classroom climate where little learning takes place (Dallman-Jones, 2006; Oehlberg, 2006).

At the other end of the behavioral spectrum, traumatized students may present with dissociation and appear very numb or passive, and as frequent daydreamers in class.

Although these students may not upset the classroom climate, they are not actively engaged in learning as they struggle with their internal fears and need for safety and control. Perry (2004) reports that, in this continuing state of fear, students hear only about half of the words spoken by teachers, causing them to fall behind year after year.

We have learned that reducing trauma-associated symptoms and behaviors improves cognitive processes and regulates children's behaviors (Fischer, 2012; Kerig & Becker, 2010; Steele et al., 2009). Helping traumatized children overcome their traumatic, sensory memories and responses to real and perceived emotional and physical threats to their well-being is the first step toward restoring learning processes and emotional and behavioral regulation. For children who are coming to school already traumatized, this help should be available where they are the most accessible—in the school setting. For those children who are exposed to school-related trauma-inducing critical incidents, intervention is also needed to prevent PTSD from taking hold of their lives and negatively impacting their ability to learn and behave appropriately. This can be achieved by immediately attending to their reactions to that critical incident and the immediate needs resulting from that experience.

Meeting Our Immediate Needs When in Crisis

Exposure to any unexpected and overwhelming situation that occurs to ourselves, the ones we love, or to our friends or peers can leave us in crisis. In crisis we prepare for the worst, experience unfamiliar emotions, and can find it difficult to think or to know what to do. The question becomes, "What do we need to do to take ourselves out of that crisis state before it also becomes traumatic?" Imagine that a loved one is going into major surgery. The doctor informs us that he will be notifying us at 3 P.M. to let us know how our loved one is doing following the surgery. We have been sitting in the waiting room for a couple of hours and then decide to go to the cafeteria or take a walk, as there are about two hours remaining before the surgery is to be completed. We return to the waiting room at about 2 P.M. because we want to be sure not to miss the doctor. Time goes by very slowly. At one point we look at our watch and it's now 3 P.M. but there still is no doctor. We again check our watch 10 minutes later, but there still is no doctor. We reassure ourselves that surgeries never start on time and that everything is going to be okay. However, we look at our watch again, and it is now 3:20 and still no doctor. Despite what we try to tell ourselves, our anxiety soars, and we worry that something may have gone wrong. It is now 3:30, and still there is no doctor. For all practical purposes, we are now in crisis, because all we can do is wait helplessly and worry.

What do we need more than anything else in this situation? We need that person in authority, in this case the doctor, to approach us in a way that immediately lets us know, without words being spoken, that everything is okay. We need to then hear the doctor provide us with the information that everything is fine and inform us as to what's going to happen over the next several hours and days. We need to know how we can reach the doctor or his informed associate in case we have questions, because in our anxiety we may have only heard half of what the doctor said to us in the waiting room. However, not until we see our loved one do we finally feel in control of that situation.

Even though it may be difficult to see our loved one lying there in a hospital bed, we begin to feel better because we are with our loved one, and can now be in a helpful role by making sure that the nurses and doctors provide the care that is needed. We call other family members and friends to let them know that everything is okay, which is also helpful because of the support they provide. Before leaving the hospital that night, after what has been an emotionally exhausting day, we need to feel confident that the nursing staff is aware of our loved one's needs and will provide care as written in the doctor's orders.

The first thing the next morning, we call the hospital to see how our loved one is doing. If they do not answer, our anxiety is activated, reinforcing the need to actually see our loved one. When we arrive at the hospital and everything is fine, we then seek information as to what is going to happen next, what the doctor said, or when the doctor might arrive, so we can begin to make plans for the next several days.

This example cites those factors that should frame the type of intervention and the timelines in which they are needed to first calm and then stabilize those in crisis. Timely applied interventions, beginning with the least intense and least intrusive, are critical to preventing further escalation of that crisis state, leaving those involved more vulnerable to trauma.

Critical Intervention Timelines

The recovery protocol that schools initiate immediately following a traumatic incident can definitely minimize the crisis they all face, while also helping to prevent the adverse manifestation of PTSD in students and staff. TLC developed a series of recovery protocol and interventions framed by critical intervention timelines in order to minimize and prevent the need for *SITCAP* in the weeks and months that follow a school's tragic event. When students and staff are in a crisis, they need for those in authority (administrators, crisis team members, and teachers) to present themselves in a way that is calming and reassuring. Students then need information (classroom presentation) as to what to expect the rest of the day, to be told how they can be helpful, to understand the choices they have, to hear that their reactions are quite normal, and to be told who is available to answer their questions and provide additional support (crisis team interventions). They also need the opportunity to spend time with friends, peers, and supportive colleagues. Before leaving at the end of the school day, they need to be sure that those in charge will be doing what is necessary to help them over the next few days, especially staff

(End of Day Staff Review). In the days that follow, they need consistent, predictable, and well-organized responses from their teachers and other school staff. The following critical intervention timelines and interventions accomplish this goal:

> **Day One**: Initiate Fan Out Meeting with all staff as soon as possible (morning when possible, before students arrive), initiate crisis intervention, begin classroom presentations, conduct staff review (for staff at end of first day), conduct defusing activities for directly exposed K-fourth graders (that day)

> **Day Two and Three**: Continue crisis intervention, complete classroom presentations, hold parent/community meeting

> **Day Four**: Support group for most-exposed students, continue crisis intervention as needed, hold brief crisis team meeting to check role assignments, what each has been least prepared for, and what is needed to help each member get through the day

> **Day Five**: Staff Review with all staff to determine remaining actions and support needed

> **Second Week**: Final crisis team review

> **Fourth/Fifth Week**: Revisit participants to evaluate status and, if needed, provide additional crisis intervention, supportive resources, or referral

> **Sixth Week and Beyond**: Initiate *SITCAP*'s school-based intervention program and/ or refer to outside trauma-informed practitioner using *SITCAP*

This overview presents both protocols (initiate Fan Out Meeting) and specific interventions. Although we briefly discuss the role protocols have in supporting intervention, our primary focus is on the interventions. For example, following a critical incident that impacts a school, its students, and staff, a wide range of reactions can be anticipated. Some will experience the incident as traumatic and others will not. To assume that all those exposed to the same critical incident need the same intervention is dangerous and can actually induce anxiety-related responses that were not previously experienced. It can also intensify reactions for those who are not ready for the one-intervention-meets-all-needs approach.

Debriefing, for example, is an early intervention that has proven to be very beneficial for many people. In recent years, it has been significantly criticized as an intervention that makes matters worse for many people (ACFASP Scientific Review, 2010). Criticism is often directed at the immediate use of debriefing following exposure. TLC uses a support group process not conducted until the fourth day following the incident, in order to allow for the outcomes of less intrusive interventions to determine the need for this group intervention must be based on the demonstrated needs of students and applied at the time needed. This support group is an excellent intervention, but *any intervention used inappropriately becomes a dangerous intervention.*

In this section we examine the timelines and rationale for *SITCAP*/TLC's approach to helping students and staff, in the first 6 weeks, to recover from the emotional and psychological responses they may have experienced following a critical incident. The timelines and interventions recommended are the result of 23 years of successful practice working in school settings with children who have been exposed to suicide, homicide, other acts of violence, the sudden accidental death of staff or students, or catastrophic events directly impacting the school and its students. These timelines and interventions are grounded in the core principles and processes of *SITCAP* programs. However, before focusing on those interventions, we want to say a few words about the importance of initiating structured protocol.

A Word About Protocol

Our purpose is not to review standardized protocol following critical incidents, but we do want to stress the importance of protocol in helping to prevent unnecessary, intense, and prolonged reactions in staff and students. An example of a protocol immediately following a critical incident would be the initiation of a Fan Out Meeting to bring all staff together before students enter the building. Intervention addresses the interaction that then takes place with staff at this meeting in efforts to best prepare them for all of the possibilities they may face when students arrive at the building (see Appendix C).

The protocols that schools immediately initiate are critical to recovery and diminishing the need for more intensive intervention. Protocol must be primarily directed at restoring and keeping all students and staff physically safe and well informed. Protocol must help staff understand their roles and responsibilities during the crisis, mobilize crisis team members to be available to help students and staff with emotional and psychological reactions in the first few days, and maintain open communication with parents and the school community. In a Fan Out Meeting, for example, we recommend giving staff a Behavioral Referral List (Carlton, Markowitz, Hadow, & Steele, 2011) that they can use as a guide to determine which students should to be referred to the crisis team for possible help (see Appendix C). Without such a guide, teachers may not recognize those who are in need, because they do not recognize a particular behavior as an indication that a student may be struggling. The longer children in need go unattended, the greater the risk is of them developing more intense reactions or challenging behaviors. This is a simple, yet very helpful protocol for reducing the emotional, psychological, and behavioral risk that can emerge for those who were still in crisis when left unattended.

Texting Protocol

In our work with thousands of school crisis team members, staff, and students dealing with critical incidents in the past 23 years, we have found that *when the simplest of protocols are not followed, emotional and psychological reactions are both intensified and prolonged.* One modern-day example of this is administrative protocol initiated following a student death. It is recommended that administrators provide an immediate response to their staff, students, and parents. We've always recommended that this response and the protocol for its delivery be drafted well before a critical incident occurs. "A time of crisis is not conducive to improvisation. Prior preparation and orientation of staff members regarding management of a crisis will greatly assist those expected to assume leadership roles and initiate actions appropriate to the time of need" (Webb, 1986, p. 476).

In today's world, staff and students will be texting each other, friends, parents, and colleagues within seconds of that critical incident. When administration fails to quickly send their message out about their awareness, readiness, and ability to manage the situation, then staff and students alike, because they are in crisis, interpret this to mean that administration is not prepared, that they will be of little help, or in some situations that they are simply not supportive of their emotional and psychological needs during such a difficult time. Even a well-crafted response delivered 30 minutes after students and staff have already been made aware of what happened will be reacted to negatively. In today's world, the administrative response needs to be as immediate as the response of those staff and students who are already texting and communicating with one another. *One inappropriately applied protocol or the absence of an organized response only adds to the crisis.*

A Protocol That Supports Immediate Needs

When people have been critically injured following a critical incident, they generally are not concerned about their emotional state. They are concerned about the extent of their injuries, the long-term impact the injuries may cause them, who will care for them or for their family while they are recovering, and how they will manage financially. To suggest in the first or second day that they must talk about their emotional reactions to what happened in order to feel better is in essence over-intervening, making erroneous assumptions as to how people may be experiencing their world, and indirectly saying, "You will get worse if you don't talk about your emotional reactions." This is for all practical purposes secondary victimization, and it directly contradicts what neuroscience and research have discovered about resilience, grief, and trauma. It is also in direct opposition to *SITCAP*'s core principles and evidence-based research regarding helping those who are experiencing grief and/or trauma.

In a crisis situation, we want a very structured approach. We want to begin with the least intrusive intervention, one that does not make assumptions but rather informs, demonstrates support, offers help to those who may want that additional support, and gives students and staff the time needed to determine how each will manage.

Begin With the Least Intrusive Response: The First Three Days

Having made the distinction between protocols and interventions, we need to ask, "What interventions do we apply when?" The first three days is the time to focus on meeting the basic needs of students and staff who have been impacted and giving them time to process and manage their reactions to this shocking, unexpected incident. All too often we simply do not give people the time or space to process their reactions or the opportunity to call on their resilience. This is one of the major criticisms of debriefing when it is applied in the first two days.

What people in crisis need initially is (a) help meeting their basic needs for safety and sense of control or choice, which needs to be integrated into the immediate administrative recovery protocol that staff are to follow, (b) comforting and supportive connections (crisis intervention) until they indicate they can manage their reactions or their reactions and behaviors indicate the need for additional interventions, (c) normalization of their reactions (classroom presentation), (d) defusing or support for the most exposed, and (e) school-based trauma interventions (*SITCAP*).

Protocol manuals need to be extensive to cover all of the possibilities that can take place in school settings. Those protocols are designed to immediately restore safety, and only after safety is established do protocols address the recovery needs of students and staff. As stated earlier, this chapter focuses only on recovery interventions, as a discussion on safety protocol would consume another book. TLC's published protocol manual is titled *Traumatic Event Crisis Intervention Plan* (TECIP). (Several examples of its protocol can be found in the Appendix C). Our discussions will then begin by examining crisis intervention followed by classroom presentations, defusing, staff review, and support for the most exposed.

Crisis Intervention: First Several Days

Following a critical incident, a wide variety of reactions will be experienced. Some may be trauma specific or cited as acute stress reactions, whereas others may reflect generalized anxiety and or grief reactions, such as worry, shock, numbness, and disbelief. A wide range of physiological reactions will also be experienced, such as crying, agitation, wandering about aimlessly, needing to leave the site, needing to talk, or being unable to talk. Crisis intervention is the appropriate intervention in the first few days, but we want that crisis intervention to be framed within a trauma-informed context.

Crisis Intervention: Promoting Resilience and Resolution in Troubled Times presents excellent intervention strategies (Echterling, Presbury, & McKee, 2005). We have worked very closely with Dr. Echterling, the primary author of this detailed description of crisis intervention strategies that are trauma informed, who supports the integration of sensory- and cognitive-based responses to people in crisis who may also be in trauma. Appropriate crisis intervention is designed to meet the basic needs of people in crisis and then help them discover that they have the strength and resilience to cope with what they have experienced. This also involves helping people to regulate their emotional and physiological reactions.

The very first chapter of the aforementioned text is titled "Resilience and Transcendence: Surviving Crisis, Thriving in Life." The authors state that all too often we focus on those in crisis as victims, and that focusing on only the victims can blind us to the survivors. The entire model is based on entering the individual's world by being curious and allowing what is learned about how students are now experiencing their world and what matters most to them to determine what we provide them at the time. This supports the primary process used in all *SITCAP* programs.

In training, we ask participants to identify all of the reactions they can anticipate from students and staff who have been exposed to a critical incident. We then take one reaction and ask participants to identify a minimum of five different ways they could possibly respond to that one reaction. When we solicit their responses, we develop an extensive list of responses that may help students to process and begin to regulate their reactions. If we take the very common reaction of crying, participants often list the following possible responses: provide a tissue, provide a glass of water, normalize their reactions, sit quietly with students, verbalize that they are now safe and can have as much time as needed to work through their reactions, ask students who they would like to be with and facilitate that connection if possible, ask who they might like to call and again facilitating that if possible, assist students with finding a quiet place so they can express themselves without worrying about what others might think about them. These are basic sensory interventions that support basic needs and regulation of reactions.

We would also ask some very basic questions to see if, despite their emotional responses, they can begin to cognitively process what they have been exposed to that day. Examples of questions might include:

➢ What might I do to help you?
➢ What do you think we could do to help others?

When students' answers are specific in their content, they are indicating to us that they can begin to process their experiences at a cognitive level. If they cannot answer these questions, they are still in their limbic region and need continued sensory-based interventions rather than cognitive-based intervention. Once they are able to engage their cognitive processes, questions over the next several days are designed to help them manage their emotions and behaviors, take action, move from victim thinking to survivor thinking, and, in time, make meaning out of their experience.

Classroom Presentation: First/Second/Third Day

Presenting a classroom announcement of what happened is different from conducting a classroom presentation. The purpose of the announcement is to empathetically inform students about what happened, to indicate that the crisis team members will be meeting with them to talk further about what happened and answer their questions, and to inform them of any changes in that day's schedule as a result of what happened. The purposes of the classroom presentation are not to process feelings, but to make an immediate connection with students, identify needs, answer questions, normalize reactions, provide helpful information, and demonstrate support. This educational intervention helps deescalate student reactions and reassures them that those in charge are managing the situation. For many students, this initial intervention is all that is needed for them to manage. Perhaps the most difficult aspect of a classroom presentation is presenting to those students who are so overwhelmed that they are unable to respond to the presenter's questions or unable to ask the presenter questions. In this case, the presenter must pose and answer the questions and concerns we know students are frequently experiencing following critical incidents. The one additional unique feature with classroom presentations is that the nature of the situation determines the kind of reactions to be normalized. For example, the reactions following suicide will be different from those following an accidental death. Presenters need to know what these differences are, and they should also be listed in the protocol manual.

What we found over the years is that when classroom presentations were not conducted, the emotional intensity of that student body was prolonged, and students felt that they were not being supported and that their responses were being minimized or ignored. Like the doctor meeting with the loved one in the waiting room, this intervention is designed to calm the anxieties and worries created by a crisis situation. On the first day following the incident, classroom presentations begin with those who are the most exposed, the classmates and peers.

Keep in mind that classroom presentations do not preclude meeting with small groups or meeting individually with the most-exposed students, who may need more attention than what can be provided in a classroom presentation. Additional classroom presentations can continue with the least-exposed students the following day. (See Appendix C for classroom presentation outline.)

Defusing

Following a critical incident, a cognitive approach is often not helpful for students in kindergarten through sixth grade who are in crisis. Defusing is an intervention that limits cognitive processing of an incident and is more appropriate for this age group. Only two basic questions are asked of nonwitnesses in defusing: (1) "What have you been told or heard about what happened?" and (2) "Since this happened, what is your biggest worry?" The two questions asked with those who were witnesses are (1) "What do you remember most about what happened?" and (2) "What is your biggest worry now?" The responses of children are normalized, rumors and exaggerations of details are clarified, and the opportunity to ask questions is presented. Following this brief cognitive focus, children are engaged in sensory-based activities designed to alleviate anxiety.

Defusing Research

We use sensory-based activities to help deactivate the arousal reactions commonly experienced by most children following exposure to critical incidents. The emotional, sensory arousal their bodies may experience simply cannot be altered through cognitive processes alone (LeDoux, 2002; Levine & Kline, 2008; Perry & Szalavitz, 2006). When younger children are helped to regulate their reactions by involving them in sensory-based activities shortly after exposure, they feel safer, less frightened, and less worried. This helps to accelerate their recovery. In one study, children explained that they learned to feel better by playing and taking part in fun activities (Alisic, Boeije, Jongmans, & Kleber, 2011). *Helping Children Feel Safe* (Steele, Malchiodi, & Kline, 2002) is a series of sensory-based experiences developed for students in kindergarten through sixth grade. These activities are designed to safely reduce children's anxiety while also empowering them with ways to regulate their fears (see Appendix B for sample activity).

Kellett (2012) reports that caregivers can help restore children's sense of emotional well-being through the use of appropriate games or other activities or by simply talking with children in a caring, supportive way. Because younger children have difficulty verbally communicating what they are experiencing emotionally and in their bodies, they need the opportunity to discharge those experiences. Children do this best by participating in safe, fun activities. Perry (2005) states that play, more than any other activity, fuels healthy developmental resilience in children. Drawing is another sensory activity, as we described in detail in Chapter 4, that helps children discharge, defuse, and manage their many reactions.

Following 9/11, the World Trade Center Children's Mural Project was unveiled on March 19, 2002. It depicted more than 3,100 portraits drawn by children. This drawing project "served to lessen feelings of isolation and helplessness felt among those children who had a hard time understanding the complexity of this tragedy" (Straussner & Phillips, 2004, p. 111). These children could not explicitly (cognitively) communicate the many ways this tragedy impacted them, but they could do so through drawing, a sensory, implicit way to communicate what words cannot. *One Minute Interventions* (Kuban, 2008) provides numerous defusing activities for all ages.

Defusing Guidelines

➤ Defusing is only for the most exposed, but because of differences in developmental needs between younger children, adolescents, and adults, we recommend initiating defusing the very first day.

> Working with younger children dictates that we remain flexible in our interventions.

> Young students fully expect the adults in their environment to be the individuals taking care of them.

> Like formal debriefing, some students will need to be followed in case this initial intervention is not helpful.

When defusing is not helpful enough, crisis intervention would be very appropriate, because it attends to several basic needs. One type of sensory support that appears unrelated to the type of the event and that can be very beneficial to the healing process, as reported by children themselves, comes from cuddly toys (Alisic, Boeije, Jongmans, & Kleber, 2008). Cuddly toys and blankies were very comforting for many children following 9/11 and are now often given to children by police, fire departments, and hospitals immediately following critical incidents. It is believed that these tangible, comforting resources bring support when parents and others are not available. These supports also come in the form of imaginary friends, which that teddy bear can become, but which may also be strictly the imaginary friends children create when tangible objects like teddy bears are not available (Henry, 2011; Taylor, 1999).

The benefits of defusing are defined by the children's response to the activities presented. If the activities are helpful, the children will quickly return to everyday behaviors. When some children continue to express their fears, they are telling us that they need additional support. Crisis intervention then becomes the next source of efforts to help them. If crisis intervention does not help over the next several weeks, a referral to *SITCAP* would be appropriate.

Staff Review

The Staff Review recommended for all staff at the end of the first day is similar to classroom presentation. The objectives are as follows:

> To evaluate the current status of staff and students/clients

> To share new information and clarify rumors

> To determine the additional need for immediate resources and support for staff and students

> To prepare staff for possible upcoming problems

> To help staff care for themselves

> To reinforce positive aspects emerging from this event

Staff Review is mandatory for all staff. Its objectives are different from debriefing for the most exposed, which is far more intrusive related to focusing on all of the details of what happened and the participants' reactions to what happened. Staff Review is directed at eliciting staff's comments, concerns, and recommendations designed to make the following day a bit easier for everybody. This process can be completed within one hour. This meeting actually gives staff a *collective voice*, which is empowering at a time when they need to feel empowered to be part of the solution, part of the recovery. By listening to their peers, it helps to unite them as a group concerned about the well-being of their students, focused on returning their school to its daily routines, and focused on reestablishing the school as a safe learning environment. When an operational debriefing is not conducted, we find that staff may not feel supported by their administration, and they may struggle with what happened and their reactions to what happened for longer periods of time.

Beyond Staff Review: Support Group for the Most Exposed

Over the years, we have provided direct services to individuals, students, and staff following such major traumatic incidents as the bombing of the Federal Building in Oklahoma City, 9/11, Hurricanes Katrina and Rita, the shooting and killing of a coach in front of students in Parkersburg, Iowa, the killing of a teacher in a school in Texas, and in far too many school situations involving suicide, violence, and sudden accidental death. Support has been helpful for most people in their efforts to regulate their reactions and care for themselves in the weeks and months that follow exposure. However, as discussed earlier, when inappropriately applied, any intervention can place participants at risk. The support group is only for the most exposed. Those most exposed consists of those who are surviving victims, direct witnesses to what happened, or are related to the victim as a family member, friend, or peer in that victim's environment. Because this process is a very formal cognitive process developmentally, it is reserved for adolescents and adults. For younger children, we use the classroom presentation, crisis intervention, and defusing activities described earlier.

The following criteria for supporting the most exposed in the school setting protects the safety of those in crisis:

➤ *Support must be voluntary.* One of the primary components of trauma-informed care is giving individuals a choice as to what they believe will be most helpful to them. To require or mandate debriefing not only places participants at risk, but also ignores the resilience research showing that many individuals do manage well with limited support. Mandating support also puts the organization or, in this case, the school at risk for litigation if the process does negatively accelerate one's reactions.

➤ *Parent permission is needed to allow adolescents to participate*, as this is a more intense intervention than crisis intervention.

➤ *This group is only for the most exposed.* The most exposed include those who were direct victims, witnesses to what happened, and/or related to the victim(s).

> *Those who are direct witnesses of the incident must be seen separately from those who are related to the victim but not witnesses to what happened.* To combine the two groups is to put nonwitnesses at risk from overexposure to the details given by witnesses.

> *Group size is important.* Group size must not exceed eight participants in order to give each participant the opportunity to respond to all the questions asked in the 2-hour time period.

> *The group must not exceed 2 hours.* To go beyond 2 hours places people, who are dealing with very frightening and sometimes overwhelming reactions, emotionally at risk.

> *At no time should those conducting the group attempt to process feelings or encourage individuals to elaborate on their feelings.* The most serious risk is approaching the process as therapy and turning the group into a treatment group by attempting to process feelings. It must be made clear that feelings are not to be processed, only normalized. People's reactions and experiences need to be acknowledged and normalized and then their thoughts shifted to how to manage the next several days and weeks.

> *The group should not be initiated until after the third day following exposure.* We must give the previous, less intrusive interventions mentioned the opportunity to be supportive while helping the majority of those exposed begin to regulate their reactions. For many, the earlier interventions will be all they need; for others, this support will also be needed.

To assume that everyone needs this support following exposure is to put people at risk of over-intervention. To conduct the group as mandatory is to ignore the needs of each individual and places people at risk from exposure they would have otherwise avoided. To allow the processing of feelings to take place turns into an at-risk therapeutic intervention at a time when people are most vulnerable and need to experience that they can manage their many emotions without having to explore them or elaborate on them.

We have found that this process of debriefing is easier to teach to nonclinical professionals. Counselors, social workers, and psychologists have often been trained to focus on exploring feelings by encouraging individuals to elaborate on their feelings and emotions. **This is not counseling.** The leader's role in our model is to ask a question and give each participant the opportunity to respond to that question. The leader does not respond to the participant's answers but simply listens. Once all participants have had the opportunity to answer that one question, the next question is proposed, and the same process is followed until all of the questions in the first two stages are completed. Before debriefing is concluded, participants' reactions are normalized, common reactions following a critical incident not mentioned are identified and normalized, and ways that participants can care for themselves over the next several days and weeks are also presented. Most will be doing well as a result of this process, but some may need additional intervention. The additional intervention may consist of brief crisis intervention or, if grief- and/or trauma-specific reactions are present, *SITCAP* would be recommended.

Keep in mind that participants represent the most exposed, those who likely have the most intense and challenging reactions because they were witnesses to the incident or closely related to the victim(s). For this reason, the final aspect of this support process is returning to participants four to six weeks later to make sure they are doing okay, to provide brief support through crisis intervention, and if needed, to refer for *SITCAP* intervention and/or to an outside trauma-informed practitioner. This is important because those who continue to have reactions are more vulnerable to PTSD. At times, participants may also have additional delayed reactions they are now experiencing.

We know that following critical incidents, some students and even staff will in fact experience a range of PTSD reactions for 6 to 8 weeks and beyond. This is when we recommend the use of *SITCAP*. It takes time to heal and recover, and the majority will when they are in an environment that is supportive, safe, and offers choice as to the help they may seek. There may also be individuals who did not participate in support efforts but six weeks or later are having delayed grief- and/or trauma-specific reactions they need help with managing. *SITCAP* is appropriate six weeks and thereafter following exposure. It is also an appropriate intervention to use at anytime during the school year with students entering school who have already been traumatized by something other than a specific school-related critical incident.

Six Weeks and Beyond: *SITCAP* in Schools

High School

What can we provide students, children, and adolescents who develop PTSD reactions six weeks after exposure to a critical incident or for those students whose PTSD preceded exposure to a school-related critical incident? Given the ratio today of counselors and social workers to large numbers of high school students attending any one school, counselors and social workers have only but a few minutes to initiate a meaningful intervention with the traumatized students to whom they are assigned. From a trauma-informed perspective, we have always believed that some intervention is better than no intervention, because it can provide traumatized adolescents with a significant connection to adults who care. In all research related to resilience and what children say helps them the most through difficult times, the number-one factor remains feeling connected to a significant adult (Brendtro et al., 2009). Studies in sociology and psychology also continually point to having at least one significant connection to an adult as the primary predictor of resilience and recovery (Bronfenbrenner, 2005). For this reason, we developed *One-Minute Interventions* (Kuban, 2008). This resource provides brief, sensory-based intervention activities when participating in the full *SITCAP* program is not available to students at school. It allows high school counselors and social workers, in the limited time available to them, to have a meaningful intervention and interaction with traumatized students that is framed by the trauma-informed practices of *SITCAP*.

One-Minute Interventions accomplishes the following:

➢ Targets the various trauma-related reactions students may be having and does so at a sensory level for reasons we have cited in earlier chapters
➢ Optimizes the interaction between counselors and students
➢ Presents students with different ways to regulate their reactions
➢ Permits counselors to maintain meaningful connections with traumatized students over time
➢ Provides students with a different way to experience themselves and their reactions, which in turn helps them to think differently about themselves, their reactions, and their ability to cope
➢ Supports students' efforts to remain resilient
➢ Provides counselors and social workers with a structured framework in which to interact with traumatized students

One-Minute Interventions affords high school counselors and social workers, the majority of whom would love to do more, the opportunity to be a meaningful adult in the lives of traumatized students. When high schools have outside resources provide their services in the school setting, we then recommend the evidence-based *SITCAP* program for at-risk and adjudicated adolescents, *SITCAP-ART*. (Examples can be found in Appendix B.)

Elementary/Middle Schools

Elementary schools have greater latitude in the ways they help their students with mental health needs. Although *One-Minute Interventions* includes activities for this age group, elementary schools tend to have the flexibility and resources to present *SITCAP*. The *I Feel Better Now!* (IFBN) program is an evidence-based *SITCAP* program used in elementary schools today. It is a group program for students 6 through 12 years of age. Middle school children may fit either the *IFBN* program or the *SITCAP-ART* program, depending on their developmental status. Both *IFBN* and the *SITCAP-ART* programs are listed on the California Clearinghouse of Evidence-Based Practices and on the Substance Abuse and Mental Health Services Administration (SAMHSA) National Registry of Evidence-Based Programs and Practices (NREPP).

IFBN Research

The original randomized, controlled study was conducted at four elementary schools. Parents whose children experienced or witnessed one or more traumatic events, as indicated on TLC Institute's Traumatic Incident Life Event Checklist, granted permission for their child to be screened for severity of trauma symptoms. The Briere Trauma Symptom Child Checklist (TSCC) (Briere, 1996) was used as the screening tool. All children with an elevated score (within the clinical range) on one of the subscales on the *TSCC* were randomly assigned to either Group A, the treatment group, which participated in the 10-week *I Feel Better Now!* program for 1 hour each week, or Group B, the waitlist or control group. After the 10-week waiting period, children and parents in Group B participated in the identical 10-week *I Feel Better Now!* program.

Three standardized trauma and mental health measures (the CAQ) were administered at pre-intervention, post-intervention, 3-month, and 6-month follow-up. Children and parents in Group B completed an additional set of measures at the end of their waitlist period. Children demonstrated remarkable statistically significant ($p < .01$) reductions in trauma symptoms across subscales of re-experiencing, avoidance, and arousal and reductions across mental health subscales including depression, somatic complaints, social problems, thought problems, attention problems, dissociation, internalizing and externalizing problems, rule-breaking behavior, and aggressive behavior (Raider et al., 2012).

Overall, the children who participated in *SITCAP*'s *I Feel Better Now!* program demonstrated statistically significant improvements, including reductions in trauma symptoms and psychological, emotional, and behavioral problems, supported by ANOVA analysis of pre-, post-, 3-month, and 6-month follow-up data of all three subscales administered. TLC's PTSD Child and Adolescent Questionnaire (CAQ) (Steele & Raider, 2001) demonstrated outstanding statistically significant ($p < .01$) reductions in all three domains of posttraumatic stress symptoms: arousal, avoidance, and re-experiencing. The Briere Trauma Symptom Child Checklist (TSCC) (Briere, 1996) demonstrated statistically significant reductions for anxiety, depression, aggression, and dissociation scales. All symptoms, as measured by the checklist, showed statistically significant ($p < .01$) reductions of trauma systems. The Achenbach's Child Behavior Checklist (CBCL) (Achenbach & Rescorla, 2001) demonstrated statistically significant improvement/reductions of symptoms and behaviors for the depression, somatic complaints, social problems, thought problems, rule-breaking behavior, aggressive behavior, activities, social interactions, and total competence scales ($p < .01$). The 3-month and 6-month follow-up data indicate maintained gains across all areas measured by the CAQ, TSCC, and CBCL. Further improvement occurred during the follow-up period in the aggressive behavior, internalizing behavior, and externalizing behavior scales, all of which showed additional statistically significant reductions. *IFBN* is a school-based program that has brought significant relief to thousands of children.

Point of Interest

Supporting Students With Special Needs Following Grief and Trauma

To provide the best support to children with special needs following grief and trauma, professionals should understand their own grief and trauma experiences, and how these experiences will impact their work. Education and training that focuses on children and adolescents with special needs, and how they experience grief and trauma, will provide professionals with hands-on, concrete techniques for intervening with grieving and/or traumatized youth with special needs.

Common mistakes when working with children with special needs following grief and trauma include the following:

- Gearing family rituals toward only those without special needs
- Not including special needs kids with special needs in grief or trauma interventions
- Lying to children with special needs or telling them half-truths about what really happened
- Using euphemisms to explain death (Grandma is sleeping, we "lost" Grandma, Grandma was sick)
- Thinking that individuals with special needs don't grieve

Following a trauma or loss, children and adolescents with special needs may exhibit symptoms and reactions such as heightened energy or exhaustion, being startled easily, heightened or decreased communication/interactions with others, regression, decreased concentration, being physically aggressive, and sensitivity to all areas of life (e.g., criticism, report card, life is unfair).

The top five things parents and professionals can do to help children with special needs following a trauma or loss include:

1. Normalize all feelings and regressions.
2. Don't just tell children they are safe, make them *feel* safe on a body/sensory level. (Safety may only be reached when modifications are made to sleeping arrangements and routines.) It should be an "all the milk and cookies you can eat" time for children.
3. Let children control what they eat, wear, and do; choose your battles!
4. Spend time *together* (e.g., play a game, read a book, look at photos, go for a walk, toss a ball, work on a puzzle). Meaningful interaction is important.
5. Greetings and goodbyes should be a big deal; make them count!

The following questions will help *identify* children's needs, which will then help direct interventions:

- What worries you the most now?
- What upsets you the most now?
- What is the worst part or hardest part for you now?
- What helps you feel a little bit better?
- What helps you feel a little safer?
- Do you have any questions about what has happened or anything anyone has said?

The progression of interventions we have discussed is beneficial when conducted in trauma-informed environments or when conducted in non-trauma-informed environments. However, gains made through these interventions are generally sustained for longer periods when the environment is trauma-informed. In Appendix D, we include several excellent resources for schools and teachers who are interested in becoming trauma-informed and engaging in trauma-informed practices. The following brief overview of what constitutes a trauma-informed environment applies not only to schools, but also to mental health centers, agencies, and programs serving traumatized children.

Trauma-Informed Schools

The volumes written about trauma-informed schools are overwhelming. Most articles identify the core principles of trauma-informed care and attempt to identify those practices that would be found in trauma-informed schools. Creating and sustaining an environment takes a well-informed and dedicated effort by everyone in that environment. In the school setting, this includes all staff and all students, as environments are not just physical places but encompass a myriad of situations that are defined by the actions, interactions, and reactions of all their members (Steele & Malchiodi, 2012).

We cannot address all of the factors that support a trauma-informed environment in this chapter, but we can briefly discuss those critical components that are rarely addressed in the literature. These components include core values and beliefs.

Core Values

The oldest and most successful childcare agencies and businesses survive because they adhere to a core set of values and beliefs (Brendtro et al., 2009; Collins, 2009; Connors & Smith, 2009). Wolin and Wolin (2000) stated, "One cannot create positive ecologies for children and youth without a unifying theme of shared beliefs and values" (p. 5). People's core values and beliefs drive their behavior. When discussing the creation of environments where children can flourish, first and foremost we need, within a trauma-informed context, to establish those values and beliefs that practice history, sociology, and psychology. If, for example, the environment does not actively pursue and support the value of respect, then a culture of disrespect develops. In a culture of disrespect, aggression, threats, and intimidation (bullying) thrive. In such a fear-driven environment, one must be chronically ready to be ridiculed, shamed, and physically attacked. People (students) in such an environment engage in primitive survival behaviors of fight, freeze, or avoidance. This environment is not conducive to learning.

Value of Respect

Focusing on the value of respect, we can understand why some classrooms are not effective learning environments. As former head of the School Psychology Division of the

American Psychological Association, Hyman documented how experiences in schools can create enduring trauma in many students (Hyman & Snook, 1999). Hyman found "that 60% of the most traumatic events reported by students were related to ridicule and mistreatment." But he was astounded to find that 40% of these destructive encounters were with school staff. For example, a student reported, "One day in Spanish class, I told the teacher I was lost and didn't know what was going on; in reply he said, 'There is a place for people like you to go to and it's called the lost and found.' The whole class laughed but to me it wasn't funny and I was embarrassed" (Brendtro et al., 2009, pp. 82–83). Practicing the value of respect can prevent further wounding of already traumatized children, as well as help children develop an appreciation of others as helpful and supportive rather than hurtful and dangerous. In such a climate of respect, students can more easily attend to and focus on learning rather than worrying and being chronically ready or aroused for the next painful attack.

Core Beliefs

What role do beliefs play in creating and sustaining an environment where children flourish and maximize their strengths and learning capacity? From a trauma-informed perspective, we believe that the child is not the problem; the environment is the problem. In other words, if the child is failing, the environment is failing the child (Bloom & Farragher, 2010). History shows that every organization that has successfully changed the lives of children in ways that allow them to flourish has a core set of beliefs that drive the behaviors of staff as well as those of the children in that environment (Brendtro et al., 2009; Steele & Malchiodi, 2012).

TLC is a program of Starr Commonwealth. Starr Commonwealth has been creating environments where children flourish for 100 years (www.starr.org/mission). One of the several core beliefs of Starr is: *We believe everyone has the responsibility to help and no one has the right to hurt anyone physically or verbally.* This single belief guides their approach to creating and sustaining an environment that is both physically and emotionally safe. It also supports the National Center for Trauma-Informed Care's (2011) primary essential focus on safety as a framework for delivering trauma-informed care. The second belief is: *We believe in recognizing and developing the strength of all children and families.* Without ever visiting Starr Commonwealth, these two core beliefs give us a very clear view of the kind of practices they must engage in, in order to create an environment that is both emotionally and physically safe and one that affords children with the opportunities to further develop and use their strengths while also discovering strengths not yet realized by them.

Another such international organization is the Circle of Courage. It integrates brain science, resilience science, and practice science to change the lives of young people across the world (Brendtro, Brokenleg, & Van Bockern, 2002). Its unifying belief is that children of all cultures have four universal growth needs: belonging, independence, mastery, and generosity. All of its practices are guided by this one unifying belief. The practices that are driven by this unifying belief were initiated in South Africa when President Nelson Mandela created a commission to transform programs for children and youth. Circle of Courage is now practiced in dozens of countries, testifying to the value of beliefs in bringing about change in children's varied environments.

Trauma-Informed Classroom Environments and Practices

Gharabagi makes two key points in his article "Reclaiming Our, Toughest, Youth" (2008). He states that, "Relationships are the intervention" (p. 31) and "Interpersonal relationships yield more than techniques (practice)" (p. 30). It is our belief that a trauma-informed classroom environment reflects the core values and beliefs we discussed earlier in this chapter. It is also our belief that the core of academic success is equivalent to the quality of the relationship that the teacher has with his or her students. To illustrate this point, we focus on the core value of respect and a belief that dictates the behavior needed to support that value.

Supporting the core value of respect in a classroom setting will evolve into trust between teacher and students because safety, choice, and value for others and their capacities are inherent in respect. Shelden, Angell, Stoner, and Roseland (2010) found that "not only was *trust* associated with greater gains in student achievement but also with lasting gains" (p. 159). The core value of respect becomes a foundation on which trauma-informed practices become successful, and that success sustained. The following strength-based, resilience-focused, trauma-informed belief supports the value of respect, allowing the classroom to become a safe environment for all students that supports their capacity to learn, and an environment that is attuned to the students' unique learning needs: *All children are capable of learning and, if they are not learning, it is not because they cannot learn; it is because we are not engaging in practices and relationships that empower them to learn.*

The following true story clearly illustrates what can happen when a teacher walks into the classroom believing in her students' capacities to learn despite what she has been told about those students. This story was made into an award-winning Hollywood movie called *The Freedom Writers*. It needs telling, because it conveys what we have been discussing about what constitutes a trauma-informed environment, as well as illustrates the transforming power of the sensory-based, trauma-informed practices we have detailed throughout this book. We, and many of the children we serve, had the honor of spending time with this inspiring teacher and individual, making her story even more meaningful and profound for us.

In 1994, Erin Gruwell, a student teacher at the time, walked into a high school classroom of 150 freshmen at Woodrow Wilson High School in Long Beach, California. Her students had already been dubbed the school rejects, and they were guaranteed to fail.

Initially, her students felt that there was no reason to be educated, as it had nothing to do with their lives. Her response was to prove her students wrong by finding ways to make her lessons speak to their experiences and, in so doing, help them tap into their talents. One of the ways she accomplished this was to help them to begin to create a journal of their experiences. As a result of their work, their collective journal became a number-one *New York Times* bestseller: *The Freedom Writers Diary: How a Teacher and 150 Teens Used Writing to Change Themselves and the World Around Them* (Filipovic, 1999). In 1998, these former "school rejects" walked across the school stage to collect their diplomas.

Practices will be of little value or meaning to traumatized and at-risk students if they are not engaged in a relationship of respect and in a relationship in which the teacher (a) believes in their capacity to learn, (b) is consistently curious about how they are experiencing life, and (c) is able to use sensory-based mediums to help them discover how their life experiences can unleash their learning capacity. Many of Gruwell's students went on to college, many are now teaching, and others are supporting the Freedom Writers Foundation. Had Erin Gruwell never respected and believed in her students' capacities, had she never given them a medium to express themselves in ways that oral language could not, neither she nor her students would have flourished.

Summary

As with participants attending our training sessions our discussions have likely raised many "What if?" questions regarding the *SITCAP* process. In Appendix A, we have listed the most frequently ask "What if?" questions and our answers to them. We hope that these will also answer the questions you may now have about the process. Before addressing what allows some traumatized children to do better than others (in the final chapter), we must first address the needs of parents of traumatized children and the use of *SITCAP* with parents. The fact is that parents of traumatized children can be traumatized by their children's experiences. We have also found that many parents of traumatized children have their own personal trauma histories, which can be activated by their children's experiences. This makes it more difficult for parents to provide the kind of support and comforting that their children need at the time. In the next chapter, we present *SITCAP*'s *Adults and Parents in Trauma* intervention program, which is designed to help parents help their traumatized children by first taking care of their own reactions to their children's trauma.

CHAPTER Eight

Interventions With Parents and Guardians

When intervening with traumatized children, their parents also frequently need varying degrees of intervention depending on their reactions to their children's trauma or the presence of their own trauma history, which is now activated by their children's experiences. In this chapter we provide a brief overview of SITCAP's (*Structured Sensory Interventions for Traumatized Children, Adolescents and Parents*) *Adults and Parents in Trauma* program. The principles and the processes used in the children and adolescent programs also provide the structure for this short-term adult intervention. Because adults are most comfortable initially with cognitive interactions, we spend more time in the initial sessions explaining the intervention processes and the reasons for them. Cognitive scripts are used to frame session activities, and as in all programs, cognitive scripts are used following sensory activities to help parents redefine the ways they think about their experiences.

After providing a narrative description of the first four sessions and several of their activities, two case examples are presented to illustrate what can matter most to parents in trauma and their concerns for their ability to best help their children. The first example is of a grandmother whose reactions to her past trauma history are activated while caring for her granddaughter. Our second example is of a young mother who was traumatized by the suicide of her husband, whose body was discovered by both herself and her two children. Without the support of an extended family, the urgency she experienced to control her reactions for the well-being of her children compelled her to seek our help.

Magical Moment

A 47-year-old woman, who experienced extreme childhood physical, sexual, and emotional abuse and suffered a traumatic brain injury at age 5 at the hands of her stepfather, began hearing voices at the age of 16. She experienced ongoing depression and anxiety and chronically abused alcohol. She frequently presented at the emergency department with suicidal ideation and suicide attempts. She was diagnosed with alcohol abuse, depression, anxiety, borderline personality disorder, and psychosis not otherwise specified (NOS).

At the time I began to work with her, she presented in crisis and was admitted to the hospital for suicidal thoughts, which she reported came from the voices in her head that told her to hurt herself. She stated there were three voices: an adult male who said mean things to her, an adult female who laughed at her, and a little girl whom she could hardly hear. She noted that not a day went by that she did not hear the voices, and the voices often got really loud and screamed at her.

There were two magical moments: First, we were sitting in her hospital room, and I asked her if she felt safe to leave. She replied: "No, I am so scared that the man will get angry with me and tell me to kill myself." For a split second I was at a loss as to how to help her. Then the magical moment came: I turned to her and said, "Well, why don't you just lock him away in a soundproof room with no windows so that you don't have to see or hear him anymore?" She replied: "Oh, I never thought of that before." I then proceeded to take her through a visual imagery exercise where we both, hand in hand, found the man, she put a room over him with no windows, then she closed the door, took the key that I gave her, and locked the door. She was instructed to give the key to me so that the woman could not convince her to open the door, because I was the one with the key. The next day she reported that she could not hear him talk, but she could hear him knocking. We then went back into the imagery, where she put a protective coating around the door to make it soundproof. Amazing! Since then she has never heard from that voice again.

The second magical moment: In case consultation, my supervisor advised against doing any form of trauma work with this woman because of her presentation and history. However, I had been using the *SITCAP* program for more than a year and a half with great success and believed that this program would be of great benefit to her. The program is safe, structured, and manageable, and it gave me the confidence, the tools, and the know-how to work safely and effectively with this woman. Psychotropic medication was utilized in conjunction with the trauma program. After the first two sessions, I could see dramatic changes, and as we continued through the program, she continued to improve and her trauma reactions diminished significantly.

I am so happy to say that for the past 8 months this woman has been doing extremely well. She has not presented to the emergency department. There have been no suicide thoughts or attempts. She no longer hears the adult male and female voices. She reports that the little girl's voice is really strong, and now when she makes reference to the voice, it is to say: "My little voice tells me it's not a good idea" as she taps her finger on her temple. She participated in and completed residential treatment for alcohol and drugs, she stopped drinking, and the nightmares and flashbacks have stopped. She no longer feels depressed. She no longer withdraws and isolates. She is reconnected with the community. She volunteers on a regular basis with several organizations. She attended a ceremony for women with hundreds of people in attendance, and she got up and gave a speech (her biggest fear was speaking out in front of people). She also plans to go back to school and has dreams of being a nurse or a counselor. She often comments: "It's strange, I feel so different, like I'm a different person!"

Even after the *SITCAP* program was completed, I repeatedly utilized the sensory exercises that further helped with flashbacks, nightmares, intrusive thoughts, images, and trauma emotions-sensations. These are the two exercises that I use. The first is to ask the individual to draw the victim and to trace it for two minutes, and the second exercise asks the person to draw their emotion, describe it, articulate what it would say if it could speak, what would you say to it if it could listen, and finally to give it a name.

Kay Noseworthy, MA, CMHC, CCC, NCC, CTS, Community Mental Health, Goose Bay, Canada

The Killing of Coach Ed Thomas

Although the program is also used with adults who are not parents, our focus will be the use of the program with parents who have experienced trauma or are traumatized by the experiences of their children. In some ways parents present more challenges because of the history they may bring with them. Their own untreated traumatic experiences are often reactivated by their child's trauma. Even parents without a past trauma history can be thrown off balance by their children's trauma and can experience significant anxiety and associated trauma reactions as a result. Several years ago in Iowa, a well-known high school football coach, Ed Thomas, was shot and killed in front of 22 of his students (Thomas, 2009). Mark Becker, one of the coach's former football players, who had been diagnosed with paranoid schizophrenia, walked into a practice session and shot the coach several times in the head. Thomas was the high school football coach for this small Iowa community for 36 years. Several of his high school players played in the National Football League (NFL). He was awarded the National High School Football Coach of the Year by the NFL, and shortly after his death he was honored with the Arthur Ashe Award of Courage ESPY (Excellence in Sports Performance Yearly) Award.

Several months later, Dr. Steele visited with school staff; they presented as a strong, resilient community, but they were still understandably experiencing a range of reactions. Later that evening, two professionals from the community and Dr. Steele met with the parents of the teens who had witnessed this horrible act of violence. The parents reported the many different reactions their teenagers were still experiencing. However, even months later, what was most prevalent was not only the level of worry and anxiety that parents had related to their sons' and daughters' reactions but also their own reactions. They were experiencing a great deal of self-doubt as to how to best manage those reactions and the reactions of their children. They were also experiencing intense fear that these reactions and those of their children would never go away.

The time allotted to spend with these parents was 2 hours. During that limited time, the reactions they described their children were experiencing were normalized, along with the worrisome, anxiety-producing reactions of the parents. Had there been the opportunity to also provide the *Adults and Parents in Trauma* program, many of the parents would have experienced additional relief. Even if these parents had no past trauma history of their own, their current reactions were understandable, but also likely keeping their children's reactions alive. This too is understandable. As is the case in smaller communities, adequate mental health resources are not always readily available or accessible. What we do know is that many of these families were supported by the strong faith practiced by this entire community. Their faith, which dictated that everyone help each other in this community, certainly supported their resilience. How then do we help parents who have been traumatized by the trauma their children experience?

SITCAP's *Adults and Parents in Trauma* Program

SITCAP's Adults and Parents in Trauma program is designed to help parents to regulate the reactions being activated by their children's traumatic experiences. When parents with their own trauma history are also activated by their children's trauma, their additional fears and worries can trigger more intense emotional reactions in their children. As parents, with or without their own trauma history, become activated, they are less able to provide a sense of emotional safety and needed comfort and soothing to their children. Regulating their reactions is even more difficult when their own earlier traumas have gone untreated. However, once parents learn ways to manage their reactions and the importance of self-regulation, they better appreciate and are able to meet the needs of their own traumatized children.

Adults and Parents in Trauma is eight sessions in length. The first three sessions are cognitive in nature but do include several strength-focused sensory activities, such as the Who I Am activity used in the children's programs but with adult-related symbols (see Appendix B for example). The information and activities we incorporate into the first three sessions allow parents to feel much safer with the process and better able to determine whether they wish to continue with the initiation of the sensory components, which include making us a witness to how they see themselves, their children, and their lives through drawing.

We review segments from the first four sessions and provide examples of one or more of the activities from each session presented. Because adults are often more comfortable and feel safer processing experiences cognitively, we provide several structured statements specific to the activity they are completing to help positively frame their thoughts about their subjective experiences.

Session One

After using handout materials to explain how the intervention process works, inclusive of empowering parents to say *yes* or *no* to whatever we ask, we normalize the reactions they are experiencing and those they may yet experience. For many parents, such as those we met following the murder of Ed Thomas, this normalizing process brings significant relief, allowing them to more easily focus on how they can be helpful to their children. *In the very first session, we indicate that it is not necessary to share the details of their experience to feel better about those experiences.* What *SITCAP* focuses on in this first session, which many practitioners unfortunately spend little time covering, is secondary victimization or wounding. The majority of trauma victims experience some degree of additional wounding weeks and months following exposure, yet rarely is this addressed sufficiently enough to help alleviate the hurt, pain, anger, self-doubt, and self-blaming that often results. We have found over the years that this one activity brings tremendous relief. Parents are deeply thankful that their exposure to secondary wounding was acknowledged and that they were given the opportunity to begin healing those wounds. Figure 8.1 shows a portion of the Secondary Wounding Checklist we ask them to complete to see the kind of wounding they experienced, as well as the extent of that wounding.

Figure 8.1 Secondary wounding checklist

Secondary Wounding	
If anyone, including doctors, nurses, police officers, social workers, clergy, or others, said any of the following to you or your child, then you have been further victimized. This may be hard to believe, because the comments may have come from people you expected to help and support you. Check all of the following comments that have been said to you or your child.	
	You are exaggerating!
	It couldn't have happened that way.
	You really can't remember that kind of detail.
	Your imagination is running away with you.
	She/he would never do that.
	There are people who have had it harder than you.
	Consider yourself lucky.
	You're still young.
	You're overreacting. You need to put this in perspective.
	What happened, happened. You don't need to be upset.
	Well, maybe if you hadn't. . . .

Reproduced with permission of TLC/Starr Global Training Network

When children, for example, have been traumatized and their behaviors remain challenging, parents are often wounded by those who see them as not taking care of their children. Victims and those caring for or related to the victims can experience secondary wounding. After parents have completed checking what applies to their experiences, we present the following framing statement:

> If any one of these statements was made to you, you have been wounded. A person's emotional "wounding" can be as difficult to recover from as severe physical wounds, often even more difficult, as it causes us to feel betrayed by those we thought would be helpful. If you checked any of these items, there is the likelihood that you experienced guilt, self-blame, and self-doubt.

We provide time for parents to discuss their reactions. The insight they gain is often very positive and focused on "No wonder I felt so bad for so long." We reframe for them how many of their reactions are not the result of the trauma or how they responded but how others responded to them following their experience. This activity becomes a very positive experience, and parents most often ask to learn more.

Always beginning and ending sessions in a safe place, we end *session one* by preparing them for what will be covered in *session two* and reframing what they have learned in this first session. Following is a brief example:

> We have covered a lot in this first session. You have learned a lot about trauma, and I have learned a lot about the ways your trauma has affected you. In the next session, I want to: Go over the results of this evaluation; talk about the ways you were victimized after your trauma; identify some additional reactions you may or may not have experienced; show you how this intervention has helped others and what they have taught us about being a survivor; and give you some ways to begin to find relief from all of this.
>
> I just want to say one more time, just as it takes time for a wound to heal, it takes time to heal from trauma. However, now that you are involved with this intervention, healing will likely be accelerated for you. After the third session, I think you will know more, begin to feel better about what happened, know whether these sessions have been enough to help, or whether you wish to continue and finish the remaining five sessions.

This framing, along with others in the session, helps to further structure the process for parents and provides a timeline for healing and encouragement that they, like others, will experience some relief. It also empowers them to let us know what will be most helpful for them.

Session Two

One of our primary efforts is to help parents focus on the fact that trauma is only one part of their lives; that many parts make them who they are today. To accomplish this goal, we use the same Who I Am activity used in the *SITCAP* programs for children. The only difference is the use of adult references in place of the child and adolescent references. The result is the same: They realize that trauma is only one part of their lives; that many parts make them who they are today. This critical activity sets the foundation for moving from *victim thinking* to *survivor thinking*.

In this session we also provide the opportunity for parents to identify and qualify other specific reactions they may be experiencing. Figure 8.2 provides a partial view of the worksheet. Thought bubbles are used to contain lists of behaviors, thoughts, and feelings associated with a specific symptom such as anxiety. The same format is used with all of the symptoms presented. Parents check those thoughts, feelings, and reactions they are experiencing, which may be related to symptoms like anxiety, worry,

Figure 8.2 Other reactions

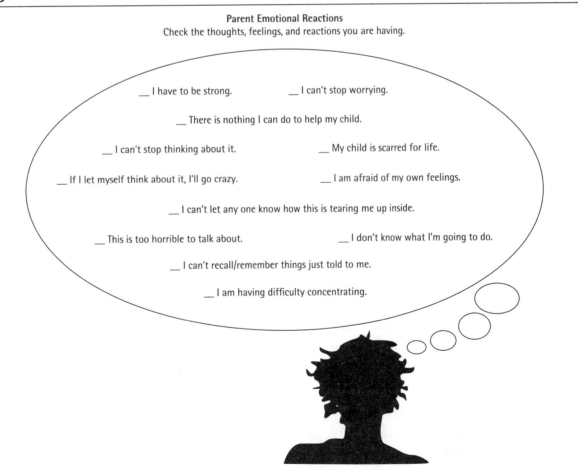

Parent Emotional Reactions
Check the thoughts, feelings, and reactions you are having.

__ I have to be strong.   __ I can't stop worrying.

__ There is nothing I can do to help my child.

__ I can't stop thinking about it.   __ My child is scarred for life.

__ If I let myself think about it, I'll go crazy.   __ I am afraid of my own feelings.

__ I can't let any one know how this is tearing me up inside.

__ This is too horrible to talk about.   __ I don't know what I'm going to do.

__ I can't recall/remember things just told to me.

__ I am having difficulty concentrating.

depression, guilt and shame, anger, and feeling powerless. This visual (activity worksheet) makes it much easier for parents to communicate their thoughts and feelings because they are there in front of them, in a concrete form, rather than being abstract reactions that are difficult to associate with specific symptoms. Over the next several sessions, they are given additional handout materials listing ways to help them better manage the most challenging symptoms. As in the children's programs, *SITCAP* interventions frequently help to reduce these symptoms.

To reinforce our belief in their resilience and ability to cope, we review with them the following framing statements. Many parents have reported during this second session that they are already experiencing one or two reactions, such as having less fear and a renewed sense of hope. These reactions are experienced, in part because of the structure of the intervention and the survivor information provided to them in these first two sessions.

As a Survivor:

➤ You will have a reduction in the number of times you experience trauma-specific reactions.

➤ You will have less fear of these reactions.

➤ You will have less fear of losing control.

➤ You will have a renewed sense of hope and direction in your life.

➤ You will redevelop a sense of humor and experience more pleasure in life.

➤ You will have a profound understanding of others' pain.

➤ You will feel stronger because of what happened and develop a new, often profound view of life.

➤ Like a wound that heals, the scar or memory will remain forever, but the pain will subside.

This activity helps create a reference for resilience and strength that can be returned to at any time the parent might become activated. As with the children's program, *SITCAP*'s sessions are structured to begin and end in a safe place to reinforce for participants their ability to self-regulate their reactions. *Session two* ends with the following reframing:

One last note here before we finish. I mentioned that trauma is only one part of your life. This is important. We are not minimizing the pain of your experience. The memory of what happened will always be there. What we are doing is diminishing the hold that experience has on you. You have been wounded deeply. It will take time to heal. When you heal, there will be a scar, in this case a memory, but the wound will no longer hurt at the level that it distracts, worries, or scares you. Your scar or memory will, in fact, in time remind you that you are a survivor, that there are other parts of you, like now, that hold your attention and are important.

Session Three

Session three provides participants with the opportunity to decide whether they wish to continue with the program. Some parents feel they can now manage, and they decide not to continue beyond this third session. We support the gains they have made and indicate that they can always call for a consultation or arrange for another appointment as needed. Although mentioned earlier, it is again important to note that, as parents discover more about trauma and their reactions to their traumatic pasts, they also begin to discover how they need to respond differently to their own children. We certainly help them with this response, but quite often they come upon this reality for themselves. Once they give their children the opportunity to express what happened and their reactions to what happened—talk less and comfort more—their children begin to experience a safer, more nurturing and protecting connection with their parents. This connection now begins to favorably alter their children's behaviors.

Unique to this session is the activity Healing Benchmarks. Figure 8.3 provides a partial list of the items available for checking at the third, sixth, and final sessions.

This activity allows parents to not only measure their progress but also see it, which is more effective than simply talking about it. Rarely do practitioners or other intervention programs allow participants to actually progressively benchmark their progress as *SITCAP* does in the third, sixth, and final sessions. The benchmarks include several statements we know participants are likely to check at the third session because of the information we have

Figure 8.3   Healing benchmarks

			Healing Benchmarks for Survivors
			You will know you are healing when you can answer "YES" to any of the following questions.
3	6	Final	
			Are you better able to understand your trauma and your reactions to it?
			Are you better able to enjoy yourself or experience pleasure more frequently now?
			Are you able to participate in activities that are important to you and bring you some satisfaction?
			Are you able to care for others?
			Are you better able to accept those trauma reactions rather than fight them or let them consume all your time and energy?
			Are you able to deal with changes in your life, even small changes, like schedules?
			Are you able to re-experience some sense of control and power in your life?
			Are you surviving?

Reproduced with permission of TLC/Starr Global Training Network

presented to them and the activities they have completed. Frequently checked are: "Are you better able to understand your trauma and your reactions to it?" and "My reactions are quite normal." This provides a visual reference to the progress being made while allowing us to indicate that healing will continue as they continue the program. Note: No matter how few or how many items the parent checks, we can provide the following comment:

In a short period of time you have learned a great deal. Just knowing what you now know has probably begun to help you in a variety of ways. You actually began healing with the first session. Although there is more we can do, you see that healing has begun.

In the remainder of the session, we spend time helping parents determine which of the suggestions listed on the program's Things To Do handout they feel they can initiate to help better manage the symptoms they are most concerned about. We clearly indicate that some may help but others may not. We add that, "Life is such that at times we have to explore several possibilities to discover which will be the best fit for us." We close out the session by returning to the Healing Benchmarks they completed to reinforce the gains they have made from working hard in each session.

Parents who have not had their own trauma history but had reactions resulting from their children's traumatic experiences will often indicate that they can manage (self-regulate) on their own now. They frequently repeat how beneficial it was to be educated about trauma, to have their reactions normalized, to hear the support and specific directions offered by the framing statements, and to not have to talk about what happened. Those who have experienced a past trauma will have similar responses but often decide to continue with the remaining program to learn how best they can manage the memories of those past reactions that their children's trauma activated. The next session is designed for those parents who wish to continue by beginning with modified drawing activities that help bring us into their past worlds to identify the influence this trauma has on the way they now see themselves and on their responses to their children.

Session Four

We include in the session the activities and trauma-specific questions associated with the major themes of trauma. As in the children's programs, the drawing activities remain structured while we remain curious. Many adults find drawing difficult, so this can be stressful, yet most report that it was of tremendous value for them, as reported in the two cases we present shortly. Knowing they will only be doing this for the one session makes it easier for them. If intervention is needed and desired following this eight-session program, then drawing provides a natural starting place for continuation and achieving a more in-depth view of their world. Following is a partial review of several of the activities and questions used with each activity in this session.

Framing the Drawing Activity

The drawing activity can be framed as follows:

> We have talked about many different aspects of your experience that have helped me appreciate what it has been like for you. The problem is that words alone simply are not enough to adequately describe what that experience was like for you. It is not the same as seeing what you see when you think about your trauma, so we are going to ask you to do a few drawings. By having the opportunity to make me a witness to how this has caused you to see yourself, others, and your life, you will no longer be alone with your experience, and it will better help both of us appreciate what may be most helpful for you. To have someone see it, the way you saw it or still see it, can bring a good deal of relief.

Creating a Safe Place

Before we begin the drawing activities, we take time to show parents what other adults have drawn and what each drawing reflected for that adult. This gives parents a reference related to how and what they can draw. The drawings presented are very primitive and drawn mostly with stick figures and one-dimensional drawings of the varied elements representing their experiences. Once parents are ready, we begin not with the trauma experience, but with a safe, pleasant memory. We frame the process in the following way:

> Before beginning with your trauma, we want you to recall some really happy time, fun time, pleasant and safe time. We will have you spend some time enjoying that memory. This will become your safe place.

We help them use all of their senses to recreate the environment where their pleasurable, fun time took place. We ask them to recall what sounds, smells, sensations of touch and taste, and what visuals were part of this fun time. We will be curious as to what they were doing that made it a fun time, who else was there, and what they were doing. Once they have spent time enjoying this memory, we present the following framing:

> As we go through the telling of your story, some memories may be emotional. If it gets to be too emotional, if you start feeling unsafe or anxious, just look at me and say "Let's stop." We will stop and give you time to go back to your pleasant, happy time until you are ready to return to what happened to you. We will call this your safe place.

We also indicate that the first 10 to 15 minutes will be the most difficult emotionally, but following this they will find some relief. When this activity is completed, we then ask them to go through the same process but now recreate the environment where the trauma took place. They are given as little or as much time as needed to recreate that moment and then told, "Whenever you are ready, I then want you to draw me a picture of what happened that you can tell me a story about."

First Drawing: What Happened

When the initial drawing is complete, we ask questions using the same curious process we detailed in Chapter 4. Examples include:

- ➤ Tell me about your drawing.
- ➤ Who are the people (names and relationship to you) in your story?
- ➤ When this first happened (if parent was a victim or witness) or when you first found out about it, what do you remember doing?
- ➤ As you look at your drawing now, is there anybody or anything not in your drawing that needs to be there? If so, go ahead and add that to your drawing.

After questions related to the drawing are completed, we then ask, "Where are you experiencing these memories the most in your body right now?" We also indicate that in just a few moments they will get some relief from the reactions they are experiencing. We listen to their answers. We want them to attend to how their body is reacting so later they can discover they have the ability to regulate their reactions by shifting to and from trauma memories and those earlier pleasant memories. This allows them to realize that they do not need to be trapped by those past memories when someone or something in their environment triggers them. We *DO NOT* begin to reflect, interpret, or try to provide insights. It is okay to ask for clarification of the details the parents have drawn or given us, but only about the information provided. If we begin to reflect and interpret, we will no longer be that curious witness.

Second Drawing: The Victim

Following this first drawing, we then ask the parents to take another sheet of paper and draw a picture of the person/victim who died, was murdered, was critically injured, left them, was taken from them, and what that person looked like at the time this happened. After completion of the drawing, a few of the questions asked include:

- ➤ As you think about it now, what scared you the most then?
- ➤ What scares you the most now?
- ➤ If that person could talk, what was said?
- ➤ What do wish would have been said by that person?

Additional questions are asked to assist the parents in describing what the experience was like. Keep in mind that the parents may take us to several different parts of their experience to help us appreciate the intensity, severity, and complexity of what that experience was like. When finished with their story for this drawing, we again ask them where they are experiencing this the most in their body and indicate that they will experience relief in just a moment.

Third Drawing: Finding Relief

In this activity we have them return to their safe place. We ask them to see it, hear it, smell it, and touch it. When they are ready, they are instructed to draw a picture of that fun time they can tell us a story about. After this drawing is completed, we ask several questions, the most important being:

> ➤ Where in your body are you experiencing this fun, happy, pleasurable experience?
> ➤ Now tell me what has happened to the trauma part?

The common responses parents give are: "It's gone," "It's not as bad," and occasionally, "It's moved." Each of these results presents the opportunity to reframe their experience. If they are no longer feeling the pain or fear associated with the drawing of what happened, then the following framing is helpful:

It is important to understand that as we went through this activity you did experience tension, but you also experienced some relief. That relief will increase in time, and I'll teach you ways to strengthen that relief. What you have learned is that you can escape those unwanted trauma reactions by returning to your safe place, changing what you think about, the way you did today. You will also learn shortly that when you simply change what you are doing you can also better manage your reactions.

Memories of your trauma experience will never go away, but now you know you can move away from those memories by going to your safe place. We will be creating several safe places for you and things you can do, so if one is not helpful at the time, you will be able to go to your other safe places or engage in those activities you will learn to use to manage those trauma reactions when they are triggered by someone or something happening in your environment.

When the outcome to this activity is "Nothing has changed," or "It's still there" (the trauma-related body response), then the following reframing is helpful:

You just learned that in the midst of your trauma memories, you can leave them and return momentarily to those fun memories, as you just experienced. The two can coexist. In time, as you are able to focus more on the pleasurable, pleasant, and fun times of your life, your reactions to those trauma reactions will diminish. It also is very likely that as we go through the remaining activities in this program, you will experience additional relief.

Final Activity: Making Meaning

The very last activity allows parents the opportunity to give their experience a new meaning, one they can manage. It also helps us discover how they are now viewing themselves and their world. In some cases, it reveals a need for continued intervention. Additional intervention often relates to family issues created by their child's trauma, family member reactions, and the need to help other family members learn ways to regulate their reactions.

The very last activity of this drawing component is for parents to put all of their drawings in front of them for one last look. It becomes another opportunity for parents to end their story in a way they can manage. Several of the questions presented are:

➤ As you look at all of the drawings, what stands out the most for you?

➤ As you look at your drawings, what surprises you the most?

➤ As you look at all of your drawings, is there anyone or anything you need to add? Go ahead and make the addition. (Ask about what was added.)

➤ Which drawing helped you the most?

➤ As you think about this now, how has this changed the way you think about yourself, others, and your world?

This last question allows us to better understand how parents reframe their thinking about trauma. It also brings them from the *then* of their experiences to the *now* of their experiences and how they will approach the future, which is often with greater resilience. This entire activity provides them with the opportunity to restructure their experiences in ways they can best manage them and make them meaningful to their life in the present. The upcoming case examples provide excellent examples of this important process. We reinforce this by having parents return to their *Who I Am* worksheets as a way to end the session focusing on the positive resources they can carry with them. We end with the following framing statement:

This was hard work today. Isn't it amazing how one terrible and tragic experience can sometimes bury and blind us to "all the parts" that make us who we are as individuals? Sometimes you just need to stop life momentarily and focus on all the good things, small or big, that have happened to you in order to reattach yourself to the many parts that make you who you are today. It is important to remember that despite all that has happened, you are a survivor. What you have learned is that, despite the tragic or terrifying incidents life has presented you, it also has given you memorable moments as well. It is important to remember that although events in your environment may reactivate those trauma memories, you can now regulate your reactions to them. You have to occasionally go back and spend time remembering these, in order to find relief from trauma-related memories. This will really help you to know that you are a survivor.

In subsequent sessions we do have parents complete a Victim Thinking Checklist and later in the program a Survivor Thinking Checklist to help them move from victim thinking to survivor thinking, which typically already began in previous sessions. They complete the Healing Benchmarks Worksheet in the sixth and the final session, and a complete session is spent on addressing their biggest worry. Using all of their activity worksheets, they also complete a *Survivor Plan* for their future, which addresses how they are now going to approach life, view themselves, their children, and others, and the behaviors they will work hard to engage that support them being not only survivors but thrivers. A detailed progression of thoughts and behaviors associated with moving from victim to survivor and survivor to thriver is presented in Chapter 9.

Magical Moment

In 1992 I had the privilege of spending time with some adult survivors of the Gulf War. In our efforts to help these survivors with the traumatic experiences they endured during this atrocious war, a mother volunteered to participate in our sensory-based process. This Kuwaiti mother was home when Iraqi soldiers invaded their home, terrorized the family, and then dragged her 14-year-old son and husband away. Her son escaped, but her husband was brutally tortured and killed.

My intervention with her took place over two sessions in two days. When asked to draw a picture of what happened, she drew a picture of her tortured husband's face and body in great detail. The details provided were quite gruesome. His body had been discovered approximately six months before I met her. From that point on, she was stuck in the horrific details of his death. Because she had drawn a picture of her husband dead, I was hoping she could draw a picture of her husband the way he looked before he was abruptly taken from her. She said she could not. She was a part of a group of eight survivors we were meeting with daily. Every day she carried with her what was referred to as the Book of Martyrs. The book contained photographs of all the tortured victims of that war in their tortured state. It included a picture of her tortured husband. She was stuck in that moment in time, unable to return to what her life was like before it happened or to move forward. Needless to say, she was having many trauma-related symptoms that were being kept alive by this constant memory of her husband's gruesome death, which she literally carried around with her daily.

The magical moment came near the end of our last session. Remember that earlier she was unable to draw a picture of what her husband looked like before he was taken away. After spending time talking about what life was like for her now, I then returned to asking her if she could now draw a picture of what her husband looked like before all this happened. She was now able to do so. I then gave her a moment to sit quietly while looking at him (her drawing of him alive) in order to say all the things she wished she could have been able to say to her husband before he was abruptly taken from her. After a moment or two of silence, she turned to us and to our surprise said she wanted to talk to him out loud. This was her way of making us witnesses to the loving relationship they shared. When she was finished, she then handed me the Book of Martyrs and said, "Thank you for returning my husband to me." What mattered most to her was to find a way to get past the horrid details of her husband's death, to return to a living memory of her husband, and to make us witnesses to the loving relationship they shared together.

This woman, as well as thousands of traumatized children and adults since then, taught us a great deal about the value of *SITCAP*, regardless of the nature of the traumatic exposures, the ethnicity of its victims, or the limited amount of time we may be given to help. The thousands of traumatized children, adolescents, and parents we have met along the way truly have been our greatest teachers, revealing what matters most, not only in healing from their terrifying experiences but also going on to flourish with a resilience many never thought possible. They really are the experts of *what matters most.*

William Steele, PsyD, MSW, TLC Founder

Practice History

Although TLC assisted many adults and parents in the early years of the program's development, its primary focus was on the development of *SITCAP* for traumatized children, as school social workers and clinicians involved in TLC were seeing far more children than parents. The realities of their environment, their responsibilities and time, and the challenges parents were experiencing in their own lives often precluded spending time with parents. When *Adults and Parents in Trauma* was formally developed in 2001, it was field-tested by 100 professionals in a variety of community settings, agencies, and programs. In addition to pre-and post-tests, field testers met for 2 full days to provide feedback related to program issues and their experiences using the program. They expressed that the amount of time given to explain to adults how the program worked, what was expected of them, the outcomes they could anticipate, and what they could expect from the practitioner was extremely appreciated and calming for parents. They further indicated that addressing secondary wounding in the very first session was extremely healing and empowering.

Most of the participating parents reported in writing that the drawing activity was hard but very necessary and helped them the most. Others cited the session on worry as one of the most helpful sessions. In essence, the session variations presented parents with multiple opportunities to experience posttraumatic growth. Although *Adults and*

Parents in Trauma never underwent formal evidence-based practice research, its pre- and post-field-testing outcomes, the testimony from field testers and the parents who participated and completed self-surveys, and its practice history supports its value. Following are two cases that illustrate *SITCAP*'s benefits even years following the original trauma.

Grandma Maddox

Grandma Maddox's story reflects the trauma parents can experience for some time following critical medical care of a newborn baby. Her drawings and story represent the kinds of sensory elements, family reactions, guilt, and self-doubt parents in similar situations can experience. These reactions can linger for years and be activated by similar situations occurring with other family members. The absence of early, trauma-informed intervention, as was the case for Grandma Maddox, may leave parents vulnerable to reactivation even years later.

The life-threatening surgery of Grandma Maddox's granddaughter suddenly reactivated the trauma that "M", who was now 50 years old, experienced some 27 years ago with the birth of her developmentally delayed son who was in a coma for 3 months. She reported that she was having flashbacks, which in fact were intrusive recollections. Her husband abandoned her shortly after their son's birth, and her mother blamed her for her grandson's condition. Her family doctor had put her on medication for depression. Appreciating that the criteria for depression and anxiety can be very similar, we initially questioned whether she was experiencing depression or anxiety.

Her pre-test outcomes indicated clinically significant levels of severity for re-experiencing, avoidance, and arousal. While still in the first session, she checked every item on the Secondary Wounding Checklist, indicating again that she had very little support from her family and that they made her feel that she was responsible for what happened to her son. She expressed that for all these years she "walked around with all these doubts" about herself, but learning about secondary wounding and seeing all the ways she was wounded, she was able to realize how her self-doubt and guilt came to be and where they came from.

When she completed the Who I Am activity in session two, she indicated, "It helped me forget a little all the bad stuff and reminded me of the things I haven't let myself do for a long time." This certainly is not the response of someone who is truly depressed. In session three she checked almost all of the items on the *Healing Benchmarks*. She indicated that she felt good about seeing her progress. At the time she asked for an index card and wrote down, "What I'm doing now reflects my best effort." This was one of the thoughts that evolved from the Healing Benchmark activity. She did not want to lose that thought, so she wrote it down and put it in her purse.

Figure 8.4   This is what happened to Grandma Maddox

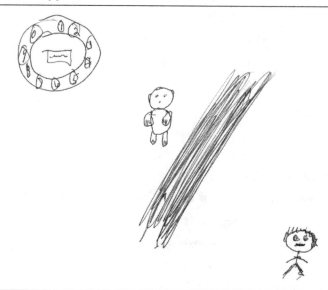

Severely activated by her granddaughter's critical surgeries, she had been in traditional talk therapy for several months with little progress. This changed quickly in *session four*, when she was asked to draw a picture she could tell us a story about (Figure 8.4).

We see in this drawing that there is a telephone on the left-hand side of the page and a baby that she identifies as a newborn at the center of the drawing. It's important to note that, in this original drawing, this newborn had no arms or hands. This aspect will become significant in the last drawing session, when she was given one last time to look at all the different parts of her story and change whatever needed changing. In the lower right-hand corner is a picture of herself far away, because she felt "so powerless not being able to be with him all the time, terrified every time the phone rang that they would tell me he died." Her son remained in a coma for 3 months. She was now experiencing these reactions once again with even greater intensity. She indicated that every time the phone rang, depicted in her drawing, she thought the worst. She also indicated that the phone represented how little support she received from family members.

When asked to draw a picture of the person who caused her so much anxiety, while her son remained in a coma, she drew a picture of her mother (Figure 8.5).

She draws the outline of her mother's face in red. As she was drawing her, Grandma Maddox's face became flushed. She began recalling some things her mother had said to her at the time, and many of these were reflected in the items she marked in the Secondary Wounding Checklist. Following this drawing, she was asked to draw what she would like to see happen to the person or thing that caused this to happen. In the

Figure 8.5   The person who caused so much anxiety

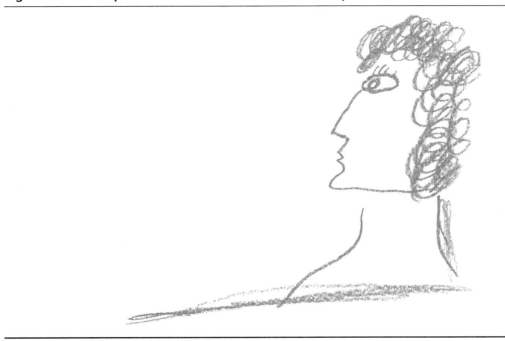

Figure 8.6   Pushing mother into tornado

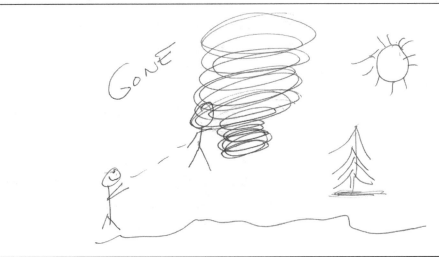

lower left-hand corner of her drawing (Figure 8.6), she indicates that she is actually pushing her out into a tornado to be taken away and never to return. (For some this is an activity they do not engage simply because there is no need for them to do so. Some have forgiven those who hurt them, while for others the circumstances are such that there is no need for anything else to happen.)

While talking about other memories related to her mother's lack of support and secondary wounding, she writes on her drawing "Gone," referring to her mother. We also see in this drawing a tree and the sun in the upper right-hand corner. The tree has much meaning for her, the significance of which we discover in the very last part of the session. At the end of this drawing, she pauses for a moment and then says, "I couldn't tell my feelings in therapy, but drawing what happened—it just clicked. It's making sense and all coming together like a puzzle."

In *session five*, which we did not describe earlier in the chapter, she was asked to check those items in the 20-item Victim Thinking Checklist that applied to her. What is important is what she does not check. What she does not check is "Most times I think things will never get better," "There is not much I can do to make my life better," and "I am never going to get over what happened to me." By not checking these three items, we are certain that when she sought our help, she was not depressed. She was more worried and anxious about her ability to manage the reactions associated with the trauma that she experienced many years earlier. After checking the Victim Thinking Checklist, she said, "It made me not like how I was, so I volunteered to be a teacher's aide." Grandma Maddox had strengths that her current anxiety and past trauma had suppressed. By being actively involved at the sensory level, she was able to rediscover these strengths.

As we were reviewing all of her drawings in the final session, she went back to her first drawing and actually added arms to the newborn that she had originally drawn. She then indicated that the newborn was really herself, but that now she was no longer helpless or feeling powerless and would be able to cope with what her granddaughter was facing. She also indicated her surprise when she saw that she had drawn her mother in red. "For all these years, I did all I could to avoid the color red because it would often make me sick. Now I know why," she said. When asked for further explanation she replied, "It was all about my mother. She loved the color red. We had lots of red in the house. When Ben (M's son) was born, she blamed me and said I shamed the family." In the drawing where she is pushing her mother into the tornado, she points to the pine tree and says, "That pine tree is me too. I am a survivor." These thoughts evolved from what she drew, not from comments we made, which is not unusual in the process when we involve parents as well as children at the sensory level. When such thoughts do emerge, reframing is almost unnecessary. Simply acknowledging M's strengths reinforced what she rediscovered about herself.

Her post-test scores indicated a 60% reduction of all symptoms across all three subcategories. Based on the many years we have used this program, we also knew that she would likely continue to see significant gains, because the intervention teaches participants a variety of ways to cope with extreme stress, as well as affords them the opportunity to now see themselves as resilient survivors. On a scale of 1 to 10, with 10 being the most severe, she rated her severity a 9 at the beginning of the program and a 3 at the last session. Most importantly, visits with her granddaughter were no longer triggering past traumatic memories, and she was more at ease with her granddaughter.

She was no longer avoiding visits but spending more time with her granddaughter doing what grandmothers do best with grandchildren—having fun, creating warm moments and fond memories.

Following the intervention she was asked what she liked most about the program. She replied, "Acknowledging I am a survivor; that I have choices." When asked what she liked least, she indicated, "Looking at all of my drawings again, but it is very necessary and I learned the most from them." When asked what the greatest improvement was for her, she replied, "I have a profound sense of freedom."

Tina's Story: Grotesque Suicide

This example is of a 26-year-old mother. One day when returning home from shopping with her 6-year-old son and 4-year-old daughter, she pulled up the driveway, stopped the car, and then got out to manually open the garage door. When she slid the door to the side, she was startled by the body of her husband hanging from the rafter. Although she reported that they had had some difficulties in the past month, she never thought he would do anything like this. Her first visit was 6 weeks after finding her husband's body. Needless to say, she remained activated and feared what this exposure would do to her children, who also saw their father hanging in the garage. She had not received treatment before beginning the *Adults and Parents in Trauma* program.

Her family doctor prescribed sleeping pills, but she said they were not helping very much. She was having panic attacks and was so frightened of the dark that she left all of the lights on in the house at night. She started to sleep with her children at night because they were having nightmares. As in all the programs, our first session spends a significant amount of time educating parents about trauma and how trauma reactions are different from grief, but also inclusive of grief reactions. When we normalized these reactions and related survivor reactions associated with the suicide of a loved one, her immediate response was, "I don't know why I get so scared, but now I know I'm not going crazy."

She checked seven statements on the Secondary Wounding Checklist, including the responses she was given by family. These included:

- ➤ "It couldn't have happened that way."
- ➤ "He would never do that."
- ➤ "There are people who have it harder than you."
- ➤ "Consider yourself lucky."
- ➤ "You're still young."
- ➤ "Well, maybe if you hadn't. . . . "
- ➤ "You should have never. . . . "

When completing this checklist, she indicated that most of the statements came from her husband's family. It was at this point she verbalized, "My husband's family never said anything to me about my pain. It was like they blamed me. Maybe this is why I am so scared, 'cause I feel like I am in this all alone."

Her pre-test scores were clinically significant in all three subcategories, with arousal symptoms being the most severe. She confirmed at the end of *session one* that she would return for the next session and indicated that what was most helpful for her was the discussion about trauma and the fact that what she was experiencing was not at all unusual, especially so soon after the suicide and given the secondary wounding she endured.

In *session two* we indicated that there may be some delayed reactions in the weeks and months to come, given all the challenges she now faced having to care for herself and her children alone. We indicated that this would not be unusual, and if the feelings were too troublesome for her, she could return for additional sessions.

She completed the Who I Am activity, circling 5 of the 36 symbols provided. Those circled reflected being sad, fearful, angry, and tired. She was not sleeping well, fearful of what the future might bring, and longing for her husband, while at the same time angry that he did what he did. We again normalized these reactions. The positive symbol she circled referenced music. When asked about this, she indicated, "I always liked my music, so I play it all night to get through the night. It seems to help my son and daughter, and sometimes I do fall asleep to it for a while." We took this opportunity to focus on the fact that trauma was only one part of her life—a big part of her life at this time, but only one part of her life. We further stated that her ability to enjoy music was indicative that, in her own time, she would be able to enjoy other parts of her life as well. We further stated that her ability to ask for help and her worry about the well-being of her children indicated that she had many strengths that would help her and her children make it through this difficult time. In response, she reiterated, "Now that I know I am not going crazy, I think I might."

In *session three* she checked one-third of the Healings Benchmarks and said, "Since the last two sessions I feel much better and know there are still hard times for us, but we will find a way to make it." She then added, "He [her husband] decided to die. I didn't want him dead. I'm going on with my life." Having worked many years with survivors of suicide, this certainly was an indication of the tremendous resilience and strength of this mother.

In *session four*, when she was asked to draw a picture of what happened, she drew a picture of her husband hanging. She provided some additional details related to how she tried to shield her children from seeing their father's "grotesque face." In the first drawing of what happened, there is no face, so she was asked to draw a picture of what his face looked like when she discovered him. In this second drawing (Figure 8.7), she

Figure 8.7   Suicide

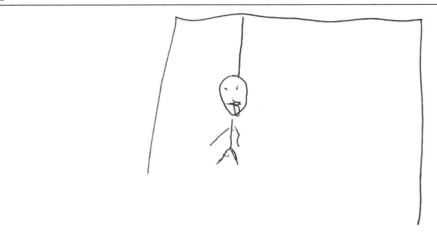

Figure 8.8   What she would like to see happen

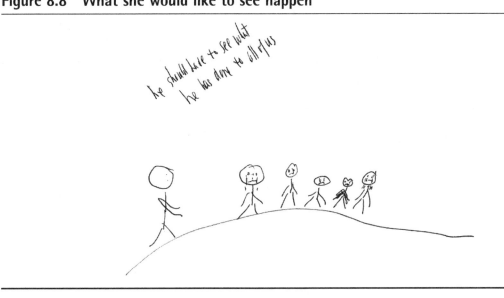

states, "His tongue was hanging out grotesquely." This was very difficult for her to do, but at the same time she reported that somehow it made it easier to talk about after she drew what his face looked like.

She was then asked to draw a picture of what her hurt or fear might look like. We see here that she draws what she referred to as a broken heart, but also writes at the bottom of the page "stupid" referring to what her husband had done, not only to himself, but also to her and her children. It often takes months—and for some survivors, years—to be able to express anger at the person who took his life. However, as she indicated, "Drawing made it easier."

The next picture she drew was what she'd like to see happen to the person who caused this pain (Figure 8.8). We see her standing in the lower left-hand corner of the page and then family members to the right, who she indicates are all crying. She wrote in the upper right-hand corner of the page: "He should have to see what he's done to all of us." However, while she shared more about what the past several weeks have been like, she then wrote in the upper right-hand corner of the page, "You can't get revenge off of a dead person." For her this was an indicator that not only was she ready to continue her life, but she was also ready to do so without being trapped by her anger, as is the case for many survivors. And, as is often the case when working at the sensory level, we were not certain what part of the intervention process helped her arrive at the conclusions she had formed at this point in the program. What is actually far more important is not the how, but that the conclusions are meaningful and a source of strength for the parent.

When she was asked what she liked most about the program, she indicated, "Drawing made it easier to talk about what happened, and it helped me believe I was okay and not crazy." When asked what she liked least about the program, she said, "It was hard to draw the pictures, but that helped me the most." And when she was asked what the greatest improvement for her had been going through the program, she replied, "I'm not so scared anymore, but I am still really angry." Following this, she reported that she no longer needed all the lights on in the house at night because she is not as afraid, and that her children were having fewer nightmares. When asked to write down any additional comments or suggestions she might have about the intervention, she wrote, "Don't change anything" and then added, "Thank you for helping me get on with living my life."

Although she had made significant progress in a short period, the worker mentioned that the challenges she could yet face in her efforts to adjust to her new life could also bring about new reactions and/or intensify the reactions, especially her anger, to all that has happened. These possibilities were normalized, as was the need to return for additional support anytime in the future. The effort with all of the *SITCAP* programs is to make the intervention process safe, so participants do feel safe about returning for additional support if and when it is needed.

Point of Interest

Repetition: What Parents Need to Know

We have learned from neuroscience that to make lasting changes in our brain, new behaviors and experiences must be repeated. This repetition allows for the formation of new neuronal connections. It is thought that new neuronal connections form quickly in children but less rapidly in traumatized children and adults.

One of the primary goals when working with traumatized children is to provide new experiences so that, with time, although previous traumatic experiences are not forgotten, the new experiences can dominate. The new experiences, when repeated, then drive the way children respond to others and situations, rather than responding in ways that are driven by older, painful experiences that have previously yielded unproductive responses. Brain chemistry changes do not happen overnight, but with repetition, they do become part of our biology.

An example of this is in the movie *The Karate Kid*. The main characters, Daniel and Mr. Miyagi, agree to work together so that Daniel can learn karate. Daniel is asked by Mr. Miyagi to do work around the karate master's house: sanding his deck, painting his fence, and waxing his cars, all in exchange for karate lessons. Before beginning, Mr. Miyagi shows Daniel specific ways to carry out each task. For example, he asks Daniel to move his hands in a certain direction as he sands. After several days of this tedious work, Daniel is frustrated and says to Mr. Miyagi, "This isn't fair. I am doing all of this work for you. When are you going to teach me karate?" Mr. Miyagi replies, "Daniel, show me, how have you been sanding the deck?" Daniel begins to make the sanding motions with his hands, and Mr. Miyagi immediately engages with Daniel to illustrate how these motions are excellent ways to block karate punches and kicks. Daniel didn't realize that as he was working, his body was engaging in repetitive motions that he now remembered without even thinking. After several months of this repetitive practice, even when under a great deal of stress at a karate tournament, Daniel's body remembered the motions, and he was successfully able to defend himself against his opponents.

When we work with traumatized children, it makes sense for us to repeatedly practice and engage with children, over and over, in activities and experiences that allow them to safely express their feelings, manage overwhelming sensations, and respond to stress as an effective way to see improvement with emotional regulation. With this repetition, over time, children will not even have to think. They will innately know how to more appropriately regulate their responses to overwhelming or stressful situations.

Summary

Given that we have now documented with research and illustrated with numerous case examples that *SITCAP* is a valued intervention for children, adolescents, and parents, we must ask ourselves what allows some traumatized individuals to do better than others. The evidence-based research outcomes of *SITCAP*'s *I Feel Better Now!* program show that all of its participants saw significant gains; these outcomes also show that, for some, even though their gains were significant, they were less significant than for the others. In the next chapter we discuss the qualitative, published research TLC conducted to determine what aspects of resilience allowed some of these traumatized individuals to do better than the others. Resilience plays a very influential role in preventing the development of PTSD, as well as assisting in determining which traumatized children may see the greatest gains. We also discover what attributes are needed to flourish by those who may see fewer gains. We identify those attributes, how they are integrated into *SITCAP*, and how they support the development of posttraumatic growth following trauma. In looking at these resilience attributes, we also identify those cognitive, emotional, and behavioral benchmarks that identify children's progressions from victims to survivors to a flourishing thrivers.

CHAPTER Nine

Nurturing Resilience and Posttraumatic Growth

The attributes of resilience provide a framework for identifying those children who are likely to be able to "bounce back" following a traumatic experience. In this chapter we identify the common attributes associated with resilience. We also examine the kinds of learning experiences that lead to resilience, and in so doing, review what our research reveals about why some traumatized children do better than others. However, this chapter also provides a review of posttraumatic growth (PTG). Posttraumatic growth defines those children with PTSD who may have had limited resilience, yet experience growth following trauma. Children with limited resilience will initially need the interventions detailed in Chapter 7—crisis intervention and they will also likely need more trauma-specific interventions like *SITCAP (Structured Sensory Interventions for Traumatized Children, Adolescents and Parents)*.

Because our primary focus is on assisting children who are traumatized, our emphasis is on the interventions that help promote PTG in these children. This growth necessitates interventions that alter the subjective experiences of traumatized children and is best developed in trauma-informed environments where trauma-informed relationships support the qualitative interactions and opportunities reviewed in this chapter. Trauma integration is the outcome of finding a balance between mind-body functions and processes, which allow us to successfully adapt to our varied environments and relationships and their challenges and opportunities. We conclude with the journey of Michelle, who, after multiple traumas, with the help of *SITCAP* and a trauma-informed environment, experiences an adaptive integration that supports her posttraumatic growth and a resilience that allowed her to flourish.

A Bounce–Back Spirit

Dr. Echterling, Professor of Graduate Psychology and Director of Counseling Psychology at James Madison University, has spent a significant amount of time with trauma survivors immediately following catastrophic situations, as well as months and years later. He has many stories to tell about the amazing resilience of survivors. While working with survivors of landmine explosions in Kurdistan, Jordan, Yemen, Iraq, and Lebanon, he provided a wonderful example of resilience. One of the survivors asserted, "I am not a victim of a landmine. The landmine is a victim of me. I survived, the landmine didn't" (Steele & Malchiodi, 2012). The spirit of this survivor is truly amazing and begs the question, "Where did that resilient spirit come from?" Resilience is frequently described as the ability to bounce back. However, if we have not been given opportunities to learn how to bounce back, doing so after trauma takes additional support. Resilience has also been described as the ability to approach life as a gift to be treasured each day, despite the crises and losses that can be experienced as part of life. However, we again have to wonder how such a view of life is developed.

For example, 9-year-old Gunnar has suffered severe, painful ear canal infections since infancy. Swimming, even with earplugs, usually brings on another infection, followed by pain from the infection, as well as the eardrops that cause him to cry before they are applied because they "burn so bad." Despite the pain he knows will follow, Gunnar jumps into the pool with his earplugs and a special rubber cap made to cover his ears and swims until dark. We again have to ask ourselves how some individuals come to develop such a resilient response, whereas others do not? What we do know is that when our losses and crises are also traumatic, they can overwhelm our core strength, beliefs, and resources.

Preventing Trauma and Encouraging Growth After Trauma
Resilience

Bonanno, Wortman, and Nesse (2004) report that individuals possessing characteristics of resilience before exposure to trauma experience initial acute stress-like reactions and, with very little support, often never develop PTSD. Punamäki, Qouta, Miller, and El-Sarra (2011), for example, found that many children living in war zones, who are faced with daily terror, violence, and poverty, constructively adapt to these situations. Morris, Shakespeare-Finch, and Scott (2007) found that resilient individuals may experience challenges in functioning capacity following a traumatic experience, but overall they have the capacity for healthy functioning and adaptation, including seeing the positive aspects derived from the experience. Betancourt and Kahn (2008) also found that many children of war find protective processes leading to resilience.

According to Cloitre, Morin, and Linares (2004), the psychological and emotional attributes associated with resilience in children include:

> ➤ Above-average verbal skills
> ➤ Cognitive and problem-solving abilities
> ➤ Positive self-esteem
> ➤ A value for others
> ➤ Ability to self-regulate behavior (bounce back)
> ➤ Positive expectations about the future
> ➤ The ability to ask for help
> ➤ Willingness to use social support

Others, like Newman (2004), describe resilient children as those who resist adversity, manage to cope with uncertainty, and are able to recover successfully from trauma. Several psychological factors also contribute to how well children adapt to stressful and traumatic events. These factors include the way children view and engage the world, the availability and quality of social resources and support, and the presence of specific coping strategies (Stien & Kendall, 2004).

We do know that resilience is learned (Ginsburg, 2006). Brooks and Goldstein (2012), Yellin (2012), Werner and Smith (2001), and numerous other sources (see Appendix D) cite various ways in which children learn to become resilient. Their greatest teachers are the adults in their lives, their parents, guardians, related family members, teachers, and so many others. The following list is just a few of the ways to teach children resilience:

➤ Being empathetic
➤ Treating children in ways that make them feel special
➤ Teaching responsibility, compassion, and generosity
➤ Infusing hope and patience
➤ Introducing children to stories of those who overcame major challenges
➤ Encouraging interest in making mistakes while providing a physically and emotionally safe environment in which to explore and take risks
➤ Recognizing strengths and deficits
➤ Providing opportunities to build strengths
➤ Identifying and reinforcing areas of competence
➤ Teaching children to problem solve and discover choices that are available to them
➤ Remaining calm when children are anxious and stressed

In essence, resilient children, when exposed to situations that become traumatic for other less-resilient children, shake it off and move forward. In fact, research demonstrates that children who use a repressive coping style (refusal to talk about what happened) tend to have fewer psychological and somatic symptoms and fewer health problems than others who do not use repressive coping (Coifman, Bonanno, Ray, & Gross, 2007; Kashdan, 2011; Weinberger, 1990; Weinberger, Schwartz, & Davidson, 1979). However, when the kinds of resilience attributes we describe are not available to children, or when repressive coping is not helpful in adjusting to terrifying and overwhelming situations, growth is halted. Reactions often become traumatic, resulting in the need for trauma-specific intervention that fosters resilience and posttraumatic growth.

Posttraumatic Growth

Turner and Cox (2004) and Tedeschi, Park, and Calhoun (1998) agree, as do we (Steele et al., 2009), that PTG is best achieved through developing a narrative and meaningful reframing of children's experiences. When they are given support grounded in trauma-informed care, many children can experience PTG and develop resilient characteristics that minimize their vulnerability when faced with ongoing or future trauma (Levine, Laufer, Hamama-Raz, Stein, & Solomon, 2008; Solomon & Dekel, 2007; Steele & Kuban, 2011). The attributes associated with PTG (Calhoun & Tedeschi, 2006; Levine et al., 2008) include:

> - Increased compassion and empathy for others (a value for others)
> - Greater psychological and emotional maturity when compared to related peers
> - Ability to self-regulate behavior
> - Increased resilience and ability to flourish (bounce back)
> - A greater appreciation for life and others
> - A deeper spiritual focus that values others and community (value for others, use of social support)
> - A deeper purpose and meaning in life (positive expectations)

These are the attributes of those who have been given the opportunity to engage in experiences that favorably change their view of self, others, and their lives. If you recall, we believe that experiences shape our thoughts (private logic), and our thoughts drive our behaviors. Affording traumatized children the opportunity to experience themselves and their traumatic experiences in a safe and empowering way reshapes the way they now see themselves and their lives, so not only are the related trauma reactions diminished, but a strength-based, resilience-focused view of self and life emerge to promote PTG.

The *SITCAP* process provides a necessary intervention leading to PTG. *SITCAP* helps children develop their narratives and meaningfully reframe their experiences. However, it also uses very structured sensory activities to alter the subjective experiences of traumatized children in ways that allow that meaningful reframing to be the result of what they experience, not what we tell them. This is the means to being able to internalize what they learn and integrate it into behaviors that now reflect the attributes of PTG. We have significantly documented the PTG-related outcomes of *SITCAP* throughout the text. We also appreciate that some children do better than others, or realize greater growth than others. All of the children who participated in *SITCAP*'s *I Feel Better Now!* research, for example, saw statistically significant reduction of PTSD symptoms and related mental health symptoms. From this perspective, they may not have had the inner resilience to prevent the development of PTSD-related symptoms, but they certainly had the capacity to change and grow. All children were also exposed to similar and multiple traumatic experiences. However, the results also showed that although all children saw significant gains, some did see fewer gains than others. This caused us to ask, "What allowed some of these children to do better than other children who participated in the *I Feel Better Now!* program?"

Interactions Influencing Posttraumatic Growth

Given that all children participating in *SITCAP*'s *I Feel Better Now!* program presented with clinically significant PTSD and related mental health symptoms following exposure to similar traumas (Raider et al., 2012), we initiated qualitative research with the children, their parents, and the social workers participating in the *I Feel Better Now!* program, to identify those experiences children had before our intervention that might distinguish differences between those who did well and those who did not do as well.

The Qualitative Study

Child, parent, and social worker focus groups were held upon completion of the 6-month follow-up period of the *I Feel Better Now!* program. Children and parents were questioned, facilitated by sensory-based activities presented in a guide given to each child and parent. For example, children were asked to rate how much their parents have helped them to feel better about scary memories by circling a specific graphic on a worksheet. The graphics were designed to represent the extent to which their parents have helped them. The categories included: a lot, a good amount, a little bit, not at all. The following graphics were included: the world, a house, an ant, and the number zero. Parents were also given worksheets containing clip art graphics created to depict several activities in which their children may participate. They were asked to select and discuss the clip art pictures that best represented their child. The parents were also asked to respond to questions verbally. Every child and parent focus group was transcribed verbatim by a court reporter.

Focus Group Observations

The following selected tables illustrate some of the most significant differences in responses between those who saw the greatest gains versus those who saw the least gains. It is important to keep in mind that those who saw the least gains overall still demonstrated significant gains in areas similar to the group who saw the greatest gains. For example, both groups reported having fewer nightmares, not being as jumpy and nervous, having less anger, and laughing more. The responses show the majority in each group. All focus group participants were given equal opportunities to participate in the discussion. Each participant was asked the same questions, and careful attention was given to prevent any group participant from monopolizing or influencing the focus group discussion.

If we simply read the different responses of the two groups of children to questions about their parents (Table 9.1), we see a much better quality of interaction between

Table 9.1   Differences Between Groups with Greatest and Least Gains

Greatest Gains	Least Gains
Better quality of interaction with parents	Absence of parental support
How much have your parents helped you feel better?	
"A lot"	"Not at all," "A little bit"
How did they help you feel better?	
"Spending time together"	"Do not help at all"
"Helping with homework"	(Majority were unable to say how their parents helped)
"Playing games together"	

children and parents of the group who saw the most gains versus the group who saw fewer gains.

The children who saw fewer gains clearly indicated the absence of support from their parent/caregiver. Furthermore, those who saw the greatest gains reported very specific interactions with parents, compared to those who saw fewer gains being unable to describe specific helping interactions. This also suggests that a very limited sense of connection and belonging existed for these children. We might conclude that these children do not see themselves as being valued as much as the children who saw the greatest gains.

The children who saw the greatest gains reported far more verbal affirmations (Table 9.2). Those who saw fewer gains reported only the one affirmation, "I love you," or "They buy me things," versus providing multiple verbal affirmations. Connections via verbal interactions were limited among those who saw fewer gains. Also, the quality of interaction that does exist is less self-enhancing and self-esteem building. Saying "I love you" is not the same as "You make me laugh" and "You are smart."

The fact that the children who saw fewer gains did not specifically identify a parent, teacher, or another adult as being important to them readily supports the absence of human connection (Table 9.3). Having a connection with someone other than a parent is frequently cited as the most significant resilience factor in the literature (Brendtro et al., 2009; Bronfenbrenner, 2005; Ginsburg, 2006; Osofsky, 2004).

A few of the children's responses, who did less well, further illustrate this absence: "My grandma, but she is dead," "I don't know, myself?" and "My parents, they have to take care of me." Not only are these children not being "treated special," but they are void of feeling really important to somebody. Children who lack connection will alienate

Table 9.2   Support From Parents in the Two Groups

Greatest Gains	Least Gains
Specific interaction with parents results in greater sense of self-worth.	Unable to describe specific interaction with parents. Limited sense of self-worth.
What are some things your parents say that make you feel good about yourself?	
"I love you"	"They buy me things"
"You make me laugh"	"I love you"
"You are smart"	
"They ask if I'm okay"	

Table 9.3   Who Is Most Important to You and What Makes You Like Them the Best?

Greatest Gains	Least Gains
Who is most important to you and what makes you like them best?	
"Parent/Caregiver/Grandparent/Uncle"	"I don't know"
"They treat me special"	"My mom"
"We play games on the weekend"	"She buys me things"

Reproduced with permission of TLC/Starr Global Training Network

Table 9.4 Parent Observations

Parent Observations	Greatest Gains	Least Gains
Improved self-esteem	86%	64%
Child talks more, more open with feelings	93%	50%
Sleeping better	71%	64%
No more nightmares	50%	50%
Less anger	71%	71%
Fewer arguments	71%	64%
Better grades	64%	50%
Not as nervous, jumpy, anxious	71%	64%

themselves and engage in avoidant behaviors. Not knowing and experiencing valued connections, they will find it difficult and threatening to trust or engage others and explore new activities. These children will have fewer peers who like them, and they will be less likely to seek help and less likely to talk to others about their difficulties.

Additional questions were asked in the original study that supported the importance of connections and the quality of interactions with adults. However, despite the differences between those who did well and those who did less well, which could be considered predictors of greater or lesser growth, parent observations (Table 9.4) indicate that even those who did less well still saw significant gains from intervention.

Promoting Resilience and Posttraumatic Growth

To improve the resilience and capacity for growth of traumatized children, we would focus intervention beyond *SITCAP* on improving child and parent/guardian/other significant adult interactions, knowing that the quality of connections children experience is key to resilience and growth (Gil, 2003; Laursen, 2008). Realizing that accessing and educating adults presents many challenges, we must keep in mind that teachers have tremendous influence in shaping children's resilience and growth because of their daily contact with children.

Teachers

More than any institution except the family, schools can provide the environment and conditions that foster resiliency (Rankin & Gilligan, 2004). Teachers are the most frequently encountered positive role models outside of the circle of family members that children encounter (Werner, 1989). Caring relationships often develop between a student and a teacher. For the resilient child, a special teacher is not just an instructor for academic skills, but also a confident and positive model for personal identification (Werner & Smith, 1992). Walsh (2012) argues that teachers, because of their daily contact with children, are often the first line of assistance for children in building resilience. Positive and caring student-teacher relationships are essential following a trauma experience, which when not present often leaves children and their families more at risk and vulnerable.

Jeang Lee (2007) found that teachers who offer trustworthiness, sincere interest, and individual attention, and who use rituals and traditions in the classroom, are often the determining factor for whether a child opens his or her mind to learn. When you show genuine interest not only in academics but also in your students' other interests, such as sports or hobbies, you are helping to improve their self-worth. When you provide a safe and positive learning environment along with setting high, yet achievable, academic and social expectations, you provide them with security and respect (Bryk & Schneider, 2002). Bickart and Wolin (1997) identified seven key classroom-teaching strategies that promote resiliency:

1. Involving students in assessing their own work and setting goals for themselves
2. Involving students in developing standards for their work
3. Offering students many opportunities to work cooperatively
4. Having students participate in classroom meetings to solve classroom problems
5. Providing children with opportunities to make choices
6. Organizing the classroom as a community and promoting student bonding to that community
7. Encouraging students to play an active role in setting rules for classroom life

It is difficult to find a single positive indicator of society's health that is not positively related to interconnectedness (Hoover-Dempsey et al., 2001). As a result of the *I Feel Better Now!* research outcomes, we developed *A Time for Resilience* (Kuban, 2009), which provides teachers and other professionals with a variety of activities to foster resilience. Students who feel they are part of their school and are treated fairly are more emotionally healthy and less inclined toward drug and alcohol abuse, suicidal thoughts, and attempts and involvement in violence (Catalano & Hawkins, 1996). When presenting to teachers (we also recommended the same for parents and other adults in the child's life), we ask them to think about the following points to reinforce the importance of creating meaningful connections with their students:

➢ Think about how exciting it is when you get a call from a friend or family member you haven't heard from for some time. It feels great to know others are thinking of you.
➢ Think about how helpful it is to pick up the phone and call someone you know just to talk. It feels great to have someone who listens.
➢ Think about how much more fun it is to attend some event with a friend or family member rather than alone.
➢ Think about how nice it is to be at some gathering and have someone come up and comment on how glad they are to see you, or how good you look.

With all that teachers have to do in the classroom to meet the standards and expectations of school districts and state guidelines, asking them to focus on building stronger connections can sound a bit overwhelming. However, there are simple ways that we can promote and foster resilience in students. The following activity is just one of several presented in *A Time for Resilience.*

Directions:

1. At the beginning of the school year (or even now) make a list of all the kids in your classroom (and school!) using the worksheet provided.
2. Next, obtain pictures of all students.
3. Place the student's name above his or her picture, and post the worksheets in the gymnasium, cafeteria, or classroom.
4. Invite all staff to come and look at the names and pictures of your students.
5. Instruct each staff member to place a sticker or checkmark next to each child's name/picture with whom they have a connection.
6. After every staff member participates, look at the names and pictures of your students. Collect all of the names of students with no (or very few) connections.
7. Then, assign two or three other teachers or staff members to make a connection with those students each week. The connection can be as simple as saying hello to them, greeting them by name, and asking how their day is going. The goal is that those students with the fewest connections experience multiple connections in school. Those adults can be any staff member, including lunchroom workers, secretary staff, other teachers, counselors, maintenance crew, and so on.

This activity was presented to us by Roger Klein (Klein & Klein, 2011), a school psychologist and one of our Certified Trainers, who understood the role connections play in creating a supportive learning environment for students and in reducing the disciplinary actions that are often associated with students who lack meaningful connections. In Appendix D we list several resources for teachers on ways to create resilient classrooms and students.

Environmental, Social, and Economic Factors Impacting Resilience and Growth

Although they are far more difficult to change, when attempting to build resilience, we would hope to address a few of the other environmental, social, and economic differences that emerged in our qualitative study and that are supported in the literature (CDC, 2011). The majority of parents of the children who saw the greatest gains were employed and had health insurance. Most were able to take their children to visit special places. Most had computers, and parents monitored their use. The children of this group, therefore, had greater opportunities for growth. Many of the parents whose children saw fewer gains were receiving public assistance, had histories of drug abuse, had unsteady employment, had mental illnesses, worked afternoons, had no medical insurance, had no computers, were unable to afford to put children in outside-of-school activities such as Boys and Girls Clubs, and/or they lived in communities that had no such resources for children.

The well-known CDC Adverse Child Experiences (ACE) study (CDC, 2011) clearly supports these findings. It makes it quite clear that children without these resources often need additional help in meeting the basic universal needs of every child: belonging (connections), mastery (self-regulation), independence (view of self as a survivor), and generosity (value for life, others, and community). The study also makes it quite clear that a family's resources play a significant role in allowing children to develop resilience early in life, as well as to make significant gains following trauma.

Evidence-based *SITCAP* outcomes clearly demonstrate that gains can be made as a result of its trauma intervention, yet those gains and resulting growth are often less when children live in the environments that do not have the kinds of connections and characteristics we have identified to be associated with resilience and posttraumatic growth. These children often benefit from additional intervention that supports the development of their universal needs (Atwool, 2006; Bowlby & Winton, 1998). One such global program is the Circle of Courage, cited in Chapter 7. The Circle of Courage, along with TLC/*SITCAP*, are programs of Starr Commonwealth (www.starr.org).

Promoting Resilience and Posttraumatic Growth Through Community

Hurd and Zimmerman (2010) and Roma and Segura (2010) indicate that the positive effects of community factors such as strong, supportive networking increases the resilience of its members. Unger, Brown, Liedenburg, Cheung, and Levine (2008) also indicated that our resilience is supported by the resources in our ecology. As indicated earlier in this chapter, the children in those families who had a greater number of resources/opportunities available to them saw the greatest gains from intervention. We briefly discuss the practices of the Circle of Courage to identify what we suggest must be the essential focus of any ongoing individual or group intervention with traumatized children, beyond *SITCAP*, who have limited connections and live in environments where resources and opportunities are also limited. Children who live in communities with the opportunity to meet their universal needs, as defined by the Circle of Courage, will become more resilient than those who lack the opportunities to meet these needs.

The Circle of Courage highlights four vital signs for positive youth development: belonging, mastery, independence, and generosity. Across history, elders in indigenous societies worldwide were highly attuned to the needs of children (Bolin, 2010; Brendtro et al., 2002; Martin, 2002). A growing body of research shows that these growth needs are the foundations of resilience and positive youth development (Brendtro & Longhurst, 2005; Brendtro et al., 2009; Brokenleg, 2012; Freado, 2010; Scales & Leffert, 2004; Tate &

Copas, 2010; Van Bockern & McDonald, 2012; Werner, 2012;). The Circle of Courage pillars of belonging, mastery, independence, and generosity form the framework within which missing developmental needs can be met to create the resiliencies that promote healthy behavior and PTG. The goal in any setting where children live, work, or go to school is to meet developmental growth needs, and, if the circle is broken, to provide restorative interventions to keep the circle complete.

Meeting These Universal Needs Through *SITCAP*

We realize that creating environments that are structured to meet the universal needs of children presents many challenges, especially given the diversity of our environments today. However, this does not minimize the need and the urgency to do so, as we are raising a generation of children who are anxiety ridden and far more vulnerable to trauma than in years past, when children were far less exposed to the magnitude of today's traumatic events, such as terrorism, war, sexual predators, economic losses, foreclosures, and homelessness (Burnham, 2009). Many factors make it difficult for children, especially traumatized children and those living in the resilience-impoverished environments described earlier, to access those interventions that support their universal needs. *SITCAP* is a beginning, and as our research has shown, it is helpful in achieving some fulfillment of these needs. Following are the ways *SITCAP* addresses the universal needs of children.

Belonging/Attachment/Significance

Children who participate in *SITCAP* experience a connectedness with the practitioner as a result of the practitioner's efforts to be continuously curious about how children are actually experiencing themselves and others in their world. This connection is further strengthened when the practitioner becomes a witness to children's worlds by having them draw the iconic images that represent how they see themselves, others, and life. This new attachment then helps to facilitate a sense of significance that is critical to enhancing self-worth: "He really wants to know what my life is like, not what's wrong with it. I am important to someone."

Mastery/Achievement/Competence

SITCAP provides children with opportunities to learn how to regulate their reactions to extreme stress as well as to reframe their cognitive understanding of themselves and life, not as victims but as survivors. Children achieve freedom from the terror of their experiences and trauma-related private logic and, in so doing, they begin to experience a sense of competence in their ability to manage what life sends their way.

Independence/Autonomy/Power

At the very beginning of *SITCAP*, children are empowered to say *yes* or *no* to whatever is asked of them. They choose which part of their world they allow us to enter; they choose when the intervention is over. In this process, children experience independence, autonomy, and the power of their choices.

Generosity/Altruism/Virtue

At the core of generosity is empathy. In the *SITCAP* process, especially in the group programs, children quickly develop empathy for what their peers have experienced, because they too have experienced many similar reactions, such as pain and terror. This empathy is generously displayed in the support and respect they begin to provide each other. Altruism develops as they begin to value what each person has to offer to one another as survivors. They also begin to appreciate the value of developing friendships and begin to relate to each other—not as someone to be feared, but as someone who may be helpful. These admirable virtues reinforce the children's self-worth.

All of this sets the stage for *SITCAP* participants' desires to continue to make new connections, seize new opportunities, exercise their independence, engage in virtues that enhance their self-worth, and master new skills that support their view of themselves as resilient survivors. For those needing intervention beyond *SITCAP*, we strongly recommend that additional interventions be strength-based and resilience-focused and allow for repetitive experiences of belonging, mastery, independence, and generosity.

Deficit-Based and Strength-Based Thinking

As practitioners focused on promoting resilience in challenging children, it is critical that our focus is strength-based. Being strength-based suggests that the way we interact and respond to children is rooted in the way we think about children who are challenging. When children exhibit extremely challenging behaviors and emotions, as is often the case with multiply traumatized children, deficit thinking often becomes more prevalent. Deficit thinking can be considered as our response to not understanding children, because we are unable to fix or control their behavior. Deficit thinking can have its roots in our own history, how we were raised, what we were taught, and how we were trained. Being trauma-informed dictates that we engage in strength-based thinking, which actually has its roots in positive psychology.

Reframing Our Thinking

Positive psychology originated from Maslow's (1954) work but did not come into its own as a new era of practice until 1998, with the help of Martin Seligman (1990), who is considered the father of the positive psychology movement. However, the First Annual Conference on Positive Psychology did not take place until 2002, and it only became an international focus in 2009, when the First World Congress on Positive Psychology was convened. Given that the focus on strengths remains relatively new, it is no surprise that deficit thinking continues in many settings and with many practitioners who were

Table 9.5   Strength–Based Versus Deficit–Based Thinking

Deficit-Based Thinking	Strength-Based Thinking
What's wrong with him?	What's right with him?
He's just a bad kid.	There is no such thing as a bad kid.
Look at his behavior.	Look at his pain.
He doesn't want to be helped.	He doesn't want to hurt.
He can't be trusted.	He needs positive adults he can trust.
He is poisoning the environment.	The environment is hurting him.
Give him an inch; he'll take a mile.	Give him a chance, and he could go far.
We know how to deal with him.	Only he knows what he's dealing with inside.
Punishment will get his attention.	Caring people will get his attention.
He needs to be knocked down a peg or two.	His own strengths can build him up.
Our policy is zero tolerance.	Our policy is positive relationships.
We have the authority.	We have his heart.
It's time to draw the line.	It's time to complete the circle.

trained by those who were trained at a time when the "allocation of attention" was on deficits, not strengths.

Finding happiness is the primary focus of positive psychology. In numerous studies related to levels of happiness, Kahneman (2011) found that the level of happiness was determined by the "allocation of attention." In essence, the greater the attention paid to our strengths, the happier we become and the more we flourish. Strength-based thinking attempts to understand what went wrong but also focuses on one's strengths to help children flourish as opposed to focusing on deficits or weaknesses. It is a shift from focusing on mental illness to focusing on mental health.

If we hope to reinforce the gains that children realize from participating in *SITCAP* or any other effort to help them become more resilient, it becomes imperative that our "allocation of attention" be strength-based. Table 9.5 compares the differences between deficit-based and strength-based thinking (Mitchell, Brendtro, Jackson, & Foltz, 2012). As we review the comparisons, we realize that strength-based thinking demands different responses, different interactions, and different views of children than the traditional deficit-based view of children. In the face of the complex challenges traumatized children can present, promoting resilience and being trauma-informed dictates that we all work hard to strengthen our strength-based thinking.

Trauma Integration

In this chapter we have listed several attributes associated with resilience and post-traumatic growth. These attributes describe how children approach and respond to life. In essence, they assist with a balanced and integrative response to life's challenges and opportunities. This is the hoped-for outcome of intervention. Rothschild (2011) states that, "Trauma treatment must regard the whole person and integrate trauma's impact on both mind and body." For example, children's abilities, as a result of intervention, to

Table 9.6   Victim–Survivor–Thriver Chart

Thriver	Resilience/ Growth
■ Life is bigger than just me now. ■ I have some new friends who are not survivors. ■ When I do think about it, I don't think about the horrid details but how it changed my life; each day is so important now. ■ The truth is I never imagined I would be doing some of the things I'm doing now, and the people I'm enjoying. ■ I enjoy having time for myself now; before I was too scared to be alone. ■ When some things happen to remind me, I now just think how fortunate I am compared to the way I was. ■ Change doesn't terrify me now, actually it's exciting at times. ■ Had all that stuff never happened, I would have never discovered how strong I am but also how important it is to have other people in my life.	■ I can control my feelings now. ■ I really am positive about my life. ■ Routines are really important to me now. ■ Now I don't hesitate to ask for help. ■ I have a lot more compassion for others. ■ I certainly appreciate life more. ■ I'm making more choices about my life than I ever did. ■ I don't ignore or shy away from problems; I go right after them until they are worked out. ■ I really try to be of help to others now. ■ Sometimes I'm even surprised by my reaction to things happening; stuff happens and I move on and it wasn't always like that. ■ I'm a lot more generous with my time.
Survivor	**Relief**
■ I no longer feel alone; I know others have had reactions like mine. ■ Things are making a bit more sense to me now. ■ It still hurts and scares me every now and then, but I'm no longer overwhelmed. ■ I can face the difficult memories head on now. ■ I am still surviving. I don't need to apologize for my behavior. ■ I am able to manage the day-to-day problems much better. ■ I hope nothing else happens, but if it does, I think I'll get through that too. ■ There are some things I look forward to now. ■ Being with other survivors I've learned I can help the new survivors coming to our group. ■ Every day isn't great, but more days are a lot better now.	■ I wake up and feel better now. ■ The hurt isn't all the time now, only when I think about before, but even that isn't too bad. ■ I remember more of what people tell me now. ■ It's easier to pay attention; I'm not as jumpy. ■ My tears don't scare me so much now. ■ I'm not so scared, period. ■ There are bad days, but the tough times don't last as long now. ■ I used to worry a lot more about bad stuff happening, but now I don't worry as much. ■ I'm sleeping a bit more; I'm even laughing a bit more. ■ I go out with friends again, a little bit more.
Victim	**Trauma**
■ I can't stop thinking about . . . ■ Everything around me reminds me of . . . ■ I'm never going to feel safe again. ■ Why even bother when I can't change a thing. ■ It's all my fault . . . I should have. . . . ■ I shouldn't have. . . . If only I had. . . . ■ It's never going to get better. ■ Why me? Why now? What next? ■ I close my eyes and see it all over again. ■ Everything makes me jump. ■ I can't think. I'm not remembering. ■ People talk to me but I can't listen. ■ I'm ready to punch anyone.	■ I think about it, see images even when I don't want to. ■ I'm afraid to. . . . ■ I worry about what next? Who next? ■ I have no energy. ■ I'm jittery. ■ I see our friend and start crying all over again. ■ I went to talk about it and started stuttering. ■ Her face, all those horrid details, they won't go away. ■ I still hear those sounds.

better regulate their responses to stressful situations improve their view of self, which leads to a more balanced response to life. Attunement with mind-body integration plays an important role in achieving this balance. Such integration also manifests itself in the form of behaviors that become proactive rather than reactive.

Assessment tools are available to evaluate levels of resilience (National Victims of Crime, 2004) and posttraumatic growth and resulting indications of integration (Tedeschi & Calhoun, 2004; Tedeschi & Kilmer, 2005). However, as practitioners we rarely see those we help beyond the intervention applied, so we may never see the full integration that takes place as the result of the path to recovery we have helped them begin. Informally, over the years, TLC has heard from children, their parents, their guardians, and those practitioners who assisted them. Their feedback and our exposure to many survivors and thrivers over the years allowed us to develop our tool for evaluating the level of integration being experienced by defining movement from victim to survivor to thriver. What we have found to be vividly descriptive as to the differences between victims, survivors, and thrivers are the different ways they experience their capabilities and express their views of themselves, others, and life. Table 9.6 depicts what traumatized children have taught us over the years about what defines them as survivors and thrivers.

We have identified some of the most frequently cited attributes of resilience and PTG and briefly discussed their relationship with trauma integration. We must also consider that being in a trauma-informed environment facilitates a greater likelihood that children will begin to learn how to bounce back, to find a balanced and integrated response to life that helps them grow after trauma. Michelle's story illustrates how *SITCAP*, combined with the trauma-informed placement where she was living, facilitated this balanced, integrated growth and resilience following her history of trauma.

Michelle's Story

Michelle's story is adapted from Steele and Malchiodi (2012). Michelle was a 16-year-old girl with a history of abuse, neglect, sexual assault, and rape. She was accepted for residential care, presenting with depression, substance abuse, difficulty paying attention in school, and verbal and physical aggression toward others. Her parents were divorced when she was very young. Michelle's abuse, neglect, and sexual assaults occurred as a child when she was living with her mother, who brought many different men into her home. She was introduced to *SITCAP* and agreed to participate.

She decided to begin by telling us the story of being raped by three boys. She was 13 years old at the time, and living with an aunt she really liked. However, during that time and up until placement, Michelle was frequently truant from school, not coming home at night, fighting with others and her aunt, and abusing various substances. Her behaviors became too difficult for her aunt, who then sought placement for her. Figure 9.1 is a drawing of what her anger was like. She colored her flames in red and orange. It was a fire she had not been able to put out, as indicated by her behaviors and symptoms.

Michelle was given several diagnoses before her placement, and at one time she was referred for psychiatric evaluation. The referral source indicated that Michelle was having

Figure 9.1   Anger

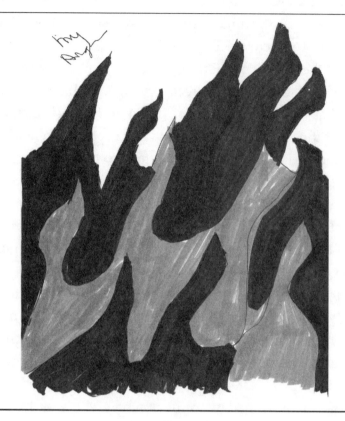

visual and auditory hallucinations. They were, as we discovered during intervention, intrusive recollections that emerged months after her rape and continued until her completion of *SITCAP*. The *SITCAP* program was recommended for Michelle because of her repeated history of trauma and unchanging behaviors. She reported that no one listened to her when she was younger. She tried to talk about what happened, but she learned that it was of no use or made matters worse, so she stopped talking (repressive coping). She also indicated that she felt tremendous guilt about the rape 3 years earlier—that it was her fault. As we tell the rest of her story, we identify that magical moment that seemed to be the turning point for her and what specifically about the *SITCAP* process was most helpful to her.

In Michelle's case, there was evidence of several resilience attributes. She had "areas of competence," especially those involving physical activities. She circled a number of the images on the Who I Am activity worksheet described earlier in the text. The images she circled reflected the enjoyment she received from playing football, playing soccer, skateboarding, fishing, and enjoying music. She had a good relationship with her father, and there were brief times she spent with him before being placed with her aunt. However, when he died suddenly from cancer, she experienced a sense of guilt for not being a better daughter. Still, she recalls very positive memories of her father.

Despite the positive connection she had with her father and the enjoyment she received from playing sports and enjoying music, she presented with clinically significant trauma and mental health–related symptoms and behaviors. A rating scale of 1 to 3 is used in the Briere Trauma Symptom Child Checklist (TSCC) described in Chapter 1. Of the 44 items on this scale, 36 were rated a 3 by Michelle, indicating she experienced the reactions checked *almost all the time* compared to 2, *lots of times*, and 1, *sometimes*. The Child Adolescent Questionnaire (CAQ) also described in Chapter 1 measures reactions within the three major subcategories of PTSD in the *DSM-IV-TR*. Her reactions were clinically significant in all three subcategories. Severity was highest for arousal, followed by reexperiencing, and then avoidance.

Providing Michelle with an opportunity to tell her story, while encouraging her to provide a visual representation of her experience by drawing, was a turning point in efforts to help her. Months of talking through her rape experience with a very caring aunt and friends and a therapist did not help. It was only when Michelle started to draw images of what happened that she had a shift in her view of self.

The trauma-specific question that helped encourage Michelle to tell her story and focus on specific details was, "Of all that has happened that brought you here today, what was the worst part for you?" Remember, what we as observers often consider as the worst part is not necessarily experienced as the worst part by the victim. Only by giving the victim the opportunity to make us a witness can we truly know the experience as he or she knows it. The use of trauma-specific questions, combined with drawing, helps provide this opportunity. When asked about the worst thing that had happened to her, Michelle clearly stated, "The rape but not the rape itself. I am an outgoing, strong girl. I was the only girl on our school football team my sophomore year—I am tough! Every day I look back and just hate myself for letting the rape happen."

By asking this one trauma-specific question, the specialist was able to help this teen work through the cognitive distortion she experienced—a focus that likely would have otherwise been missed. Michelle's view of herself was that this was all her fault, and with that came her sense of shame and view of self as, "I am no good." Keep in mind that she felt that she had disappointed her father and certainly her aunt. As a child, her mother abused and neglected her and allowed her to be used sexually. The guilt and shame of the rape included, at a sensory level, the combined sensations, visual memories, and feelings of the guilt, shame, pain, anger, and loss of empowerment she had experienced since childhood.

When asked, Michelle drew a picture of what happened (Figure 9.2). Her drawing again reminds us that we can never be certain about what we are looking at until children tell us in their own words what their drawing represents. In the upper left-hand corner is a television in an entertainment center. Directly below this is a couch with her and her two friends. Directly below that image is a depiction of a sliding-glass door and a deck where the three boys came into the house. In the upper right-hand corner are the stairs going to the bedroom, drawn below the stairs is the bed with the heads of the three boys who raped her.

Figure 9.2   What happened

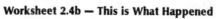

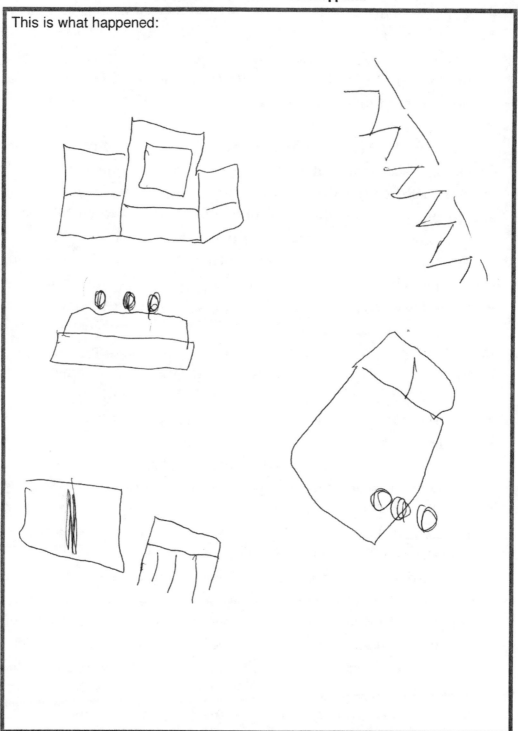

When using drawing to help children externalize their trauma memories, children will also, with the help of trauma-specific questions, begin to relate to those experiences differently once they are outside themselves in a concrete form. In Michelle's case, after drawing what happened, she sat quietly for a moment. When children actually see their experience now in a concrete form outside of themselves, as their own observers of what happened, they also sometimes begin to remember additional details that allow them to arrive at a different understanding and view of themselves. This happened for Michelle.

After looking directly at her drawing for a moment, she then looked up from that drawing and said, "I did do everything I could to try to stop the rape from happening. It wasn't my fault." That drawing provided Michelle with a visual representation that allowed her to now see and recall details that had been buried by her guilt and her shame, not only related to the rape, but also to the trauma she could not avoid as a child. What this drawing allowed her to realize that talking about her trauma did not, was that she did everything she could do to escape that situation and her earlier abuse. Others had tried to tell her it was not her fault, but only after engaging in this sensory activity could she now remember things differently and see herself in a more positive way. It also became that turning point, that magical moment, that became the beginning of her posttraumatic growth.

Michelle had indicated that she was not allowed to talk about the things that happened to her as a child while with her mother. For years she used repressive coping as a way to manage her pain. She continued to attempt to cope this way well into her teens, but her symptoms and behaviors indicated that this was not a helpful strategy. Even when she began talking to her aunt and even the therapist at her placement about all that had happened to her, it did not bring relief from the pain, guilt, and shame she had lived with for years, nor did talking about it change her behaviors. *SITCAP* intervention continued over the next several weeks, using drawings and related trauma-specific questions to help Michelle explore the many subjective experiences of the trauma she experienced throughout her life.

Figure 9.3 is a drawing that Michelle completed in the closing sessions of *SITCAP*. It reflects what we referred to earlier in the text as being the critical reframing needed to move from victim thinking to survivor thinking: *Trauma is only one part of my life; there are many parts to me that make me who I am today.* She now defines herself as "full of energy and having a heart." At the end of *SITCAP*, no items on the TSCC were rated 3, and only six items were rated a 2 (experiencing that reaction lots of times). The overall reduction of symptoms across all *DSM-IV-TR* subcategories was 90%. *SITCAP*'s practice history and evidence-based research outcomes also tell us that Michele's outcomes would have been sustained even if she were not in her current environment. The rest of her story supports the value of also being in a trauma-informed environment that provides multiple opportunities for growth.

Figure 9.3   Two parts

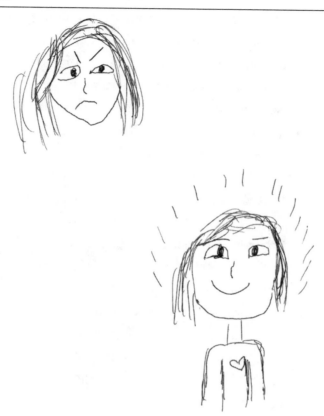

Over the three months that followed *SITCAP*, while she was still at her placement, Michelle joined the school choir and found her voice. She knew she enjoyed singing, but as she indicated, "I didn't know that I was actually good at it!" Michelle's participation in the agency choir provided her with a sense of belonging. She was part of a peer group with similar interests, many of whom she connected with immediately. After a few weeks, Michelle was practicing to sing a solo for a board member retreat. Michelle recalls the day of her performance vividly. She described in detail, "It was scary, but I just knew I could do it. As soon as I started caring about and believing in myself, I noticed that other people do too—even adults care about me," she said. "All the things I did in the past, all the bad things, well, I am bigger than that now, there is more to me than that". Singing with the choir provided Michelle with an opportunity to master one of her interests in the company of like-minded peers. Michelle was now not only in the school choir, but also a travel choir that participated in events across the country.

When Michelle was asked to provide one or two words to describe herself before she started her treatment, she indicated, "sad and ignorant." When asked to use one or two words to describe herself now, she exclaimed, "pretty amazing!" Her verbal description reflects the same significant changes indicated by the post-assessment tools and in her drawing. A more balanced and integrated response to life was now allowing Michelle to flourish.

Michelle graduated from high school just before the end of her placement. She was returned to her aunt and, after a brief stay with her aunt, she enrolled in college and began sharing an apartment with some peers. Michelle came to see herself as having value and was now able to value others as well. She developed a much deeper compassion for others and a deeper purpose in life. She went on to live an independent, autonomous life of her choice and learned to regulate her behavior. She is flourishing.

Summary

SITCAP is a resilient model and one that helps children and practitioners grow emotionally and professionally. It has a 23-year practice history and has demonstrated very successful evidence-based research outcomes. It is also framed by the major criteria establishing a practice as being trauma informed. It is a short-term intervention that produces long-term gains for children. It can be used in any setting with minimal training. Program materials are well organized and easy to use, and it provides practical, straightforward instructions and tools for implementation. Its structured format also ensures greater fidelity to its intervention processes and primary focus on maintaining the safety of the intervention for the child and the practitioner.

Essentially, it is a process that assumes that "children do not want to hurt," that "only children know what they are dealing with inside," and that we can "give them a chance to make us a witness as to how they are experiencing their world," and they will reveal *what matters most* to them while demonstrating their resilience and capacity to grow. The many traumatized children, like Michelle, who are and have participated in *SITCAP* over the years do challenge us, but they also show us their resilient spirits over and over again. The spirit they generate in us is to never stop being curious about the worlds they live in and experience every day, while we continue to respond in ways that matter the most to them.

A

What If? Questions

Participants being trained to use *SITCAP* are given every opportunity to ask questions regarding its processes. In every *SITCAP* training, participants are placed in small groups and given time to discuss the intervention model. Following this, they are instructed to write down at least one question about the process and then to submit those to us. We instruct them to begin each question with "What if?" We present, in this appendix, the most frequently asked questions presented to us over the years and our responses to them. Hopefully they include questions you may have after learning about *SITCAP*.

What If? Questions and Answers

What if the trauma just happened, when do we begin *SITCAP*?

Currently, Acute Stress reactions, as detailed in the *DSM-IV-TR* (APA, 2000), appear from the onset of the incident up to 4 weeks following the incident. Reactions of Acute Stress are the same reactions of PTSD. The only difference between the two is a period of 4 weeks. When Acute Stress reactions continue beyond a 4-week period following a traumatic incident, then the diagnosis becomes PTSD. Regarding the 4-week Acute Stress period, it is important to consider that this period can be prolonged when the trauma incident has prevented the return of the normal operating systems of one's infrastructure. This happens frequently in community tragedies, such as when floods or hurricanes take out the main roads, electricity, and water. The absence of these day-to-day support systems can prolong and sometimes intensify the reactions of Acute Stress. A prolonged delay can also increase vulnerability to PTSD.

The Developmental Trauma Disorder (van der Kolk et al., 2009), proposed for inclusion in the *DSM-5*, uses the duration criteria of 6 months following the initial exposure before assigning its diagnosis. During that 6-month period, supportive interventions and appropriate changes in the environmental conditions associated with that trauma can prove very beneficial in the prevention of PTSD and or resolution of Acute Stress reactions. The *DSM-5* (APA, 2012) has now added the new duration criteria period as 6 months, rather than 4 weeks, following initial exposure for the assignment of PTSD. We refer you to Chapter 7 for the Critical Incident Intervention Timelines discussion about which interventions are recommended during this duration period.

SITCAP has traditionally been administered any time *beyond* the first 6 weeks following exposure to trauma. The new duration criteria does not change the use of *SITCAP* 6 weeks and beyond because of its focus on the subjective experiences children are having since their exposure that are difficult for them and creating new challenges in their lives.

What if an entire family has been traumatized, how do we proceed?

Although it is very time consuming, we recommend that each member be seen individually when an entire family has been traumatized. Each member needs the opportunity to tell his or her own story, as each member will be impacted differently. Once each member has gone through this individual process, the entire family can be seen together to tell their collective stories. Remember the discussion we had about how not everyone exposed to the same situation will necessarily be traumatized and, if traumatized, the intensity of each of those reactions may differ.

To meet with the entire family following a trauma is difficult. Members simply look at one another, and the memories of what happened are triggered. It is as if they can never get away from it. This explains why, in many cases, even in the most open family systems, members will each take different roads in their attempt to avoid memories of their trauma experience.

Families have complex histories with each other. We do not want those histories to interfere with each member's opportunity to safely revisit their experience. The purpose of meeting with each individual member is to create a sense of safety that allows each person, in privacy, to revisit the way each reacted, to develop his or her story (trauma narrative), and then to reorder it (cognitive reframing) in a way that each can now manage and feel safe telling others what he or she feels safe revealing. Some may be able to accomplish this in one session, whereas others may need several sessions. The *SITCAP* programs appropriate for each age level are used for this purpose. Sessions are followed sequentially. Not everyone will need every session. Once each member has found relief, and only after each member is feeling better, does the entire family sit down together so each member can safely tell how they experienced or are experiencing that trauma.

What if siblings need *SITCAP*?

For the same reasons detailed in the answer to meeting with an entire family, meet with siblings separately. Children especially will have issues with safety. Each will want his or her own special attention. Each certainly needs to tell his or her own story, which they may not be able to do with their sibling present because of their relationship. One sibling, for example, may be more dominant than the other and not provide the less-dominant child the freedom to bring us into their world. Seeing siblings separately can prevent embellishment, duplication, and the avoidance of different reactions.

What if I am unsure whether to provide individual or group intervention? What are the differences?

With the *SITCAP* model, the only major difference between the two is the time needed. The activities and the focus on the subjective experience remains the same. The group sessions are one to two hours in length versus the 10- to 45-minute sessions for individuals based on their developmental levels. It will simply take more time for eight children to bring us into each of their worlds. The group format is actually much easier than the individual format. In the group program, members quickly normalize reactions for one another; they begin to support one another as survivors. The issue is that not all children can tolerate the stimuli of group meetings, which can be overwhelming. The absence of privacy can also induce anxiety, so for some children the individual program is safer.

It may not be discovered that children really need the safety of individual intervention until several group sessions have been conducted and they repeatedly struggle to follow very basic ground rules. The simplest of the ground rules is that only one person at a time talks while everyone listens. Some children cannot follow this ground rule because the group is too stimulating or they may lack internal control. Whenever the safety of the individual is being or about to be jeopardized, intervention is directed at restoration of that sense of safety. For some children it may mean the use of both individual and group sessions; for others it may mean movement from individual to group, or group to individual.

What if the child or children, when in a group session, simply have a lot they want to tell us and we are unable to complete the activities in that session?

Each session addresses a major theme or subjective experience. Some children, for example, will have less reaction to worry but have more issues with hurt. It may take one to two meetings to complete the activities for that session. For some it may take only 20 or 30 minutes to complete that session theme. When this takes place, we simply begin the next session. In field tests, both the individual and the group programs were completed within the time frames provided, despite the time it took to complete each session. Although *SITCAP* programs are structured, there are opportunities to spend more or less time on the various themes of trauma depending on what is most important for the child.

What if there is ongoing trauma?

Our TLC Certified Consultants and Specialists have repeatedly reported that *SITCAP* interventions have given children they work with a new resiliency, allowing them to direct their new energies to the other difficulties in their lives. *SITCAP* helps children change the way they think about and see themselves, others, and life in ways that are associated with the characteristics of survivors and resilient thrivers. This new view of self, others, and life make them less vulnerable to the ongoing stress and trauma they may be exposed to in their daily lives.

What if a child's behavior suggests trauma, but there is no history available to validate trauma exposure or the child has no memory of the trauma in his or her life?

In these situations, we recommend dealing with the child in the present. As a starting point, we suggest beginning with worry by asking, "Over this past week(s), what has been your biggest worry?" Worry is a safe place to begin with most children when no specific incident has been identified. This is a question children generally find easy to answer, which leads quite easily to addressing what has been the worst part of their present circumstances (being in foster care, school difficulties, etc.). From this point on, the full *SITCAP* program can be initiated to help them deal with their subjective experiences related to recent struggles.

Because we are addressing subjective experiences and implicit sensations and memories, we can help children gain relief even when the facts of specific incidents are not available. Even if what children are experiencing is not trauma, they still receive much-needed help to deal with their feelings in ways many others never address. How many times, for example, do we actually spend time asking children about their biggest worry, how big it is, what it looks like, if it had a name what would its name be, and what the child could do while he waits for the worry to go away? Worry contains elements of fear and anxiety. Help children with their worry, even if it is not trauma related, and we help reduce their level of anxiety. Reduce levels of anxiety, and children's ability to attend, focus, and be less reactive improves.

What if the trauma is experienced prior to age 3?

If we accept that trauma is a sensory experience first, not a cognitive one, then we accept that children younger than 3 years of age do have a sensory memory of their exposure to trauma. The October 1999 *Harvard Mental Health Letter* (vol. 16, no. 4) reviewed research on the "Neurobiological Effects of Early Trauma." It discusses, for example, that early experience can cause prolonged hypersensitivity to Acute Stress. We also know the body remembers those sensations associated with traumatic experiences even at the preverbal stage. *SITCAP* interventions are about helping children to express themselves even when words are not available or simply fail to describe what is being experienced. It is also designed to help children find relief from those body memories and sensations through nonverbal sensory activities. We recommend the *Zero to Three* (Kuban, 2009) resource of sensory activities we have available as part of the overall *SITCAP* programs when assisting infants and toddlers.

What if I am unsure who should be included in *SITCAP* programs?

Caution is urged with those having a major psychiatric diagnostic disorder such as bipolar disorder, paranoid schizophrenia, or borderline personality. Little research is available that identifies any population that should not engage in sensory-based activities. In field tests we completed *SITCAP* successively with children diagnosed with autism, elective mutism, ADHD, depression, and a host of other disorders that were also accompanied with psychotropic medications. However, research and practice history are badly needed to isolate the unique trauma intervention needs and strategies beneficial to special populations. There is still a great deal we do not know related to children. What we do know is that we must continue to challenge ourselves to seek out varied approaches to helping traumatized children.

What if someone says I am increasing the risk of retraumatizing children by having them relive their experiences?

First, we do not have the child relive his experience, but revisit it as an observer from a safe position. We empower children to say *yes* or *no* to whatever we ask. If children do not feel safe, their response to intervention is likely to be "I have nothing to tell." The *SITCAP* model is very structured and guided by the focus on maintaining the child's safety. Exposure is only the first step. We want to give that trauma a language, and take it from a sensory memory into a concrete, tangible form, which can then be reordered or reworked in a way that the child's present life view of self and others becomes manageable.

Of the thousands of interventions provided by TLC Certified Consultants and Specialists across the country, we have not had one report since 1990 of any child who was unable to return to the classroom because he was activated during *SITCAP* intervention. This is not to say it has not happened, however, because safety is always a priority and the activities inherently allow children to find their safe place if the activity becomes too difficult. The intervention is a balance between dealing with trauma memories and pleasant memories. This process empowers children to determine what is safe for them.

All sessions and activities move children from victim thinking to survivor thinking. Sessions move from the sensory to the cognitive as another way of returning to a safe place. Sessions are structured to also end in a safe place. If children were to become severely activated, we would immediately stop the intervention and engage in those sensory activities discussed and referenced throughout this text that may help deactivate their arousal while maintaining their physical safety. Thereafter, we would attempt to solicit their help to identify what triggered their reaction: Was it the activity or a delayed reaction to something that may have occurred prior to the session?

Because drawing is a major component of *SITCAP*, what if the person doesn't want to draw?

If children do not want to draw, it may be that, at a sensory level, they do not feel safe. This has to be honored. On the other hand, the initial response to not wanting to draw is often in response to not knowing what to draw or not having a reference point as to what kind of drawing effort is acceptable, for example, stick figures or full-body drawings.

Because you have spent a good deal of time already educating and normalizing trauma as part of the *SITCAP* process, the child or adolescent has likely already given you some credibility and trusts you to know what is best. Following are suggestions to make the process a bit safer or easier for those children who are not sure what to draw or how to draw it.

Children often just need a reference point to start.

If they say, "I don't know *how* to draw."

Response: "Let me show you what I mean." Draw one or two stick figures, a primitive drawing of some aspect of the child's experience, and then say, "It doesn't matter how you draw, just that you draw."

If they say, "I don't know *what* to draw."

Response: "You know sometimes there is just so much that happened we don't know where to begin. Let's try this. . . . " Ask them to just very briefly describe what was in the environment where this happened. Select one component of that environment, such as an object, and say, "Why don't you start with. . . . "

If they say, "I don't know how to draw *it*."

Response: "What is it you are thinking about drawing?" If they are wanting to draw a person but not sure how, have them begin with just one part of the person, like a circle that could represent the person's face; "Why don't you just draw a circle and that will be the face." If it is an object, start with one part of the object; "Why don't you start with a line and that will be the beginning of. . . . "

If they say, "I don't *want* to do this."

Response: "I know it's hard even being here. It certainly isn't fair that this had to happen, but it did. But you do not need to draw right now to feel better and I do want you to feel better, so how about we. . . . "

At this point we can engage in those activities that children indicate they feel okay doing at that time. Keep in mind that the relationship is the intervention, and we want children to experience us as someone who is safe, who listens, and who does help them feel safer. Also trust that, if we continue to remain curious about all that children are doing and saying, they will eventually value our suggestions of what might be helpful. We would use trauma questions to help them tell their story, if they are willing to do so, but what matters most is children's emotional safety.

What if the child doesn't want to talk?

The response "I don't want to talk about it" can be the result of several situations. Situation one refers to the child's experiences with trying to talk about the details of what happened to his parents or other adults. The details terrify the adult. Predictably, the adult says, "This is only making us feel worse. It's not helping. It's best we stop talking about it and get on with things." This is an understandable response, as exposure via details can be frightening and leave the adult frightened that they and the child will lose control. However, this response leaves children believing that adults really do not want to hear the details, so they say "no" to those who ask them to talk about it. This means that we must present ourselves as someone who is really curious to know what it has been like for them.

Situation two relates to not having words to adequately describe the experience. Even adults will have a difficult time finding words to describe their experiences. So when children are asked if they want to talk about it, they may want to, but they become anxious because they do not have the words to do so. This then causes them to shut down verbally, and that is why drawing can be so helpful when words and language are not accessible.

Situation three is related to a response that is similar to stuttering. For some children it is almost impossible to form the words. It's as if they get stuck in the throat and the vocal cords can't push them out. This response to talking about what happened would terrify anyone and easily lead to not wanting to talk about what happened. Safety again becomes critical to making this response less frightening. Drawing is a way to safely communicate what children may be afraid to verbalize or not have the words to do so.

What if the child I am working with is deficient in verbal skills? Can the initial session and other activities still be done?

Yes. There are several ways for children to communicate and for us to communicate with them. Reading *Brave Bart: A Story for Traumatized and Grieving Children* (Sheppard, 1998) can be very helpful, as can having children communicate or express themselves through puppets, drawing, and other expressive activities. Children can also provide one-word *yes* or *no* responses to questions or even nod their head in agreement or disagreement. The challenge is to remain patient and to provide children with those mediums and materials that allow them to portray what they are experiencing and for us to respond as appropriately as possible.

Children with Asperger's syndrome can have immense difficulty forming relationships; can this bring about trauma reactions in these children?

Yes. Activation and self-regulation are often a prominent focus of intervention. Everyday social situations, like walking down the school hallway to go to their classroom, for example, can be activating and cause several associated reactions. Patience and repetitive efforts to help strengthen self-regulation become a primary focus of our efforts to help children with Asperger's.

Can the sensory interventions be used with children who have been diagnosed with an autistic spectrum disorder or other pervasive development disorders? If so, do adaptations need to be made?

Yes. Adaptations will be based on the developmental levels of children. A 16-year-old in this case may developmentally do best with activities from *SITCAP*'s *I Feel Better Now!* program designed for children ages 6 through 12 years old. It is important to know that these children often have different reactions that we might otherwise consider to be inappropriate but are quite normal in their world. For example, when children in residential care are scheduled for a visit from their parent, who then cancels, they may have no reaction to not seeing that parent but have quite a different, very activating reaction, to not being able to play with their X Box. As stated throughout this text, what matters most is how children are experiencing their world. This is where we begin our efforts to be helpful.

What if I am trying to get parents involved in *SITCAP*?

Parental involvement is critical to outcome, yet obtaining parental involvement often meets with numerous barriers, some avoidable, others in part due to the challenges and trauma history of parents. TLC's programs initially limit the time involvement, yet structure sessions with parents to maximize that involvement. Typically, attendance at a minimum of two sessions is requested of parents. These sessions include the intake session and a parent-child session structured to help make the parent a witness to how the trauma has impacted their child, similar to how the intervener has become a witness. A session following the initial session with the child is optional and used to give the parent feedback about their child's evaluation results and status. Many parents will schedule this session. Some will be open to the presentation by phone, if it is not possible for them to attend.

Parents who have had a previous history of trauma and are now reexperiencing that trauma because of their children's trauma, or themselves have been traumatized recently, can find help through additional sessions available in *SITCAP*'s *Adults and Parent Trauma Intervention Program* reviewed in Chapter 8. In any case, scheduling a meeting with the children's parents or primary caregivers to provide them with an opportunity to explain their major concerns regarding their children's symptoms or behaviors is helpful and allows an opportunity for us to provide parents with some education regarding trauma and how it may be impacting their children. Education helps parents begin to make sense of their traumatized children's changes following exposure.

What if a parent/guardian is not agreeable to taking part in being a witness during the parent-child group session or individual session when the child is to use his drawings to tell his story to his parent/guardian?

Without parental involvement, the level of reduction of reactions is likely to be less than if the parent is involved. Research detailing the importance of parental involvement is abundant. If using the group program, children could be assigned a special task to assist us during that group session while the other children are telling their stories to their parents. This allows them to at least experience a connectedness with us. If their parents are simply not willing or interested in being a part of this process, it becomes paramount that the reality of what this means for those children becomes a part of the intervention before and following that session. Sensory interventions apply here as well. For example, we can explore what the worst part of this is for children, where they feel this the most in their body, and so on. Obviously this is a situation in which we would hope to spend additional time with these children until other adult connections can be made.

What if I do not follow the interventions in the sequence presented in the *SITCAP* model?

Field testing and research have shown that some sensations are safer to manage before others. Each *SITCAP* session builds a sense of safety and power that then allows the engagement of the more difficult sensations, such as anger and accountability. The outcomes documented in field testing and research are based on following the intervention sequence. This does not exclude making a decision not to use an activity based on what we know about children and the direction they are taking us.

What if I want to skip the education component of *SITCAP*?

We do not recommend skipping the education component. *SITCAP* intervention programs use specific resource materials for the educational component of the process to ensure that children have some sense regarding what they are about to experience as well as learn. Structuring statements during the intake session clearly identify how the process works, what will be expected, and what outcome can be anticipated. The difference between grief and trauma is taught to each child. Each child's trauma reactions are also normalized. This helps them to make sense out of what happened. When supporting the fact that what is being experienced is quite normal, anxiety decreases. Education also provides the tools needed to regulate trauma-specific reactions, which results in increased mastery and control over one's self.

What if I want to use activities other than drawing?

We recommend this structured intervention because it is designed for safety. It moves very slowly and helps to isolate the major troublesome areas very quickly so, should additional intervention be needed, the focus of that intervention is clear. Other methods can certainly be helpful, but we believe they are best initiated after completing *SITCAP*. *SITCAP* will clearly identify focus areas that may need pursuing using other interventions, especially expressive interventions. However, other expressive interventions tend to lack structure, which lessens the sense of safety. They may be directed by the insight or analysis of the intervener, as to what children are expressing and needing, rather than letting children identify what matters most to them. Using additional expressive interventions following *SITCAP* can be quite appropriate and extremely beneficial if they are structured to address the subjective experiences *SITCAP* reveals are in need of additional intervention. This process is one in which curiosity continues and the intervener follows the lead of the children, as detailed in the text. Given our concern that other expressive interventions be structured, we have developed several advanced sensory activities that facilitate a focus on trauma-related themes that may need additional attention.

What if someone asks me what traumatized children need the most?

The need for safety is paramount. Children of trauma have to reexperience physical and sensory safety so that the arousal response can lessen. This means not only physical safety, but a feeling of safety with self and with parents and caregivers—the ability to consistently rely on them for structure, care, and comfort. Traumatized children need to know they are not alone with their terror and grief. They need to have their feelings and reactions normalized by hearing stories and seeing the reactions of peers who were also traumatized by either violent or nonviolent traumatic incidents.

A medium for communication is essential for traumatized children, who often may not have the words to describe their experiences. Such communication mediums include playing, drawing, or storytelling to allow children to express their feelings safely. These activities come naturally to children. We can learn more of what children are feeling through these activities than by asking questions like "How do you feel?" Traumatized children need to learn that their reactions, as well as reactions they might yet experience as a result of their trauma, are normal.

The opportunity to reattach emotionally to the adult world, which they may perceive to have betrayed them by letting this trauma happen, is also important for all traumatized children. Traumatized children need to have the time and trauma-specific attention to help them find relief from their terror and to develop a sense of power over that terror. And lastly, they require the opportunity to replace that terror with happy, empowering memories.

What if there are multiple traumas. Where do I begin?

Begin with the most recent trauma or the trauma the child feels has impacted him the most. For some there have been repeated exposures to the same type of incident, such as witnessing domestic violence. For these children we recommend asking them to identify the worst time they feel stands out the most. Because TLC's trauma interventions focus on sensations rather than trauma-related behaviors, multiple traumas to some degree become irrelevant in the intervention process. Hurt is hurt. The sensation of "hurt" will reflect the sensation of "hurt" experienced across multiple traumas. This is not to say that there are not unique details to each experience that can play an important role in healing. These details may need to be pursued if intervening around the most recent trauma is not benefiting children. It has been TLC's experience, as reported by many TLC Certified Trauma Specialists and Consultants, that children do, in fact, experience relief without having to return to every trauma situation.

What if I need to determine if the child I am seeing is no longer viewing himself as a victim but as a survivor?

The following statements are reflective of individuals who think and behave as victims (Steele & Malchiodi, 2012, p. 192):

➤ I have to accept bad situations, because they are part of life, and I can do nothing to make them better.
➤ I don't expect much good to happen in my life.
➤ No one could ever love me.
➤ I am always going to feel sad, angry, depressed, and confused.
➤ There are situations at work and at home that I could do something about, but I don't have the motivation to do so.
➤ Life overwhelms me, so I prefer to be alone whenever possible.
➤ There are only a few people I can trust.
➤ I feel I have to be extra good, competent, and attractive in order to compensate for my many defects.
➤ I feel guilty for many things, even things that I know are not my fault.
➤ I feel I have to explain myself to people so that they will understand me, but sometimes I get tired of explaining and conclude it's not worth the effort, and choose to stay alone.

Thoughts of Survivors
As a survivor, I know and believe the following about myself:

➤ Yes, bad situations come up in my life, but I can do things to make them better.
➤ I expect a lot of good to happen in my life.
➤ I am loveable and people love me.
➤ I may feel sad, angry, depressed, and confused today, but I will not always feel this way. Things will get better.
➤ I have a lot to offer the world, and I am motivated to go forward.
➤ I am capable. I handle life with confidence.
➤ I can trust most people.
➤ I am a worthy person. I have many traits that are worthwhile.
➤ I am only responsible for myself. I cannot control everything.

As survivors, children will have a reduction in the number of times they experience trauma reactions. They will have less fear of these reactions and less fear of losing control. They will have a renewed sense of hope and direction in their lives, redevelop a sense of humor, and experience more pleasure in life. Children moving to survivor thinking will reestablish positive relationships with peers, adults, and family members who are supportive. They will develop a profound understanding of other people's pain. They will feel stronger because of what happened and develop a new, often profound view of life. The thoughts of survivors are far different than those of victims. In Chapter 9 we present a chart showing the progression of thoughts, behaviors, and feelings from that of a victim to a survivor to a resilient thriver.

What if the child has anger issues?

We must first remember that trauma is not a cognitive but a sensory experience. Children and adolescents experience trauma at a sensorimotor level and then shift to a perceptual representations at symbolic level. Knowing this, we begin to first work through the subjective experiences before addressing the behaviors, unless those behaviors are putting others at risk. Attempting to control those behaviors without helping to change the view children have of themselves and others is likely to be limited when the behavior is being driven by the internal trauma memories. The behaviors we see (relating to the anger) will usually be driven by how children view themselves and the world around them. When children are given the opportunity to present us with their iconic representations of themselves through drawing and other expressive mediums, we will then truly know how the trauma has impacted them, its relationship to their anger and anger-related behaviors, and what will be helpful.

What if a child has been sexually abused; do I start by asking her to draw me a picture of what happened?

Following the education process, *SITCAP* programs begin with safe activities that vary with age ranges before asking children to draw what has happened. When working with children in a group setting, conducting an individual session prior to joining the group is recommended. This session is to identify what each child does not want others to know, as well as helping each child determine what he or she is safe drawing in a group setting when it comes to that specific activity. Ideally, sexually abused children would be placed in a group with other sexually abused children.

What if we cannot provide a comprehensive trauma-informed assessment; what would we try to evaluate?

Although we did not discuss what constitutes a comprehensive trauma assessment, we recommend that a limited assessment identify children's cognitive processes, sensory integration development and trauma history including family/parent history, what activates them, and what helps to calm them. We would also want a comprehensive developmental history. (For more about our trauma assessment courses and Trauma Assessment Specialist Certification, go to www.starrtraining.org/tlc.)

What if we know a child is not relating factual information when talking about what happened?

What matters most is children's recollection of what happened to them or around them. This is their reality and what is driving their behavior. We should always stay with children's perceptions of what happened, regardless of whether those perceptions are real or imagined. Intervention is not about challenging the memory but providing new sensory-based experiences that change the way they now see themselves and their world. When this view changes, so too does their behavior.

What if a child says he is feeling better and does not want to continue the program?

As we stated earlier, trauma-informed practice supports choice. If children no longer want to continue the intervention program, indicating that they feel better now, then end the intervention, reinforcing the progress they have made. Remind them how they can return at any time. It is important to contact children in a few weeks to see how they are doing as a way to let them know we are thinking about them.

What if the child reveals abuse or some other life-threatening situation while taking part in *SITCAP*?

As in any intervention process, the duty to inform and refer does not change. (Check your state-mandated reporting laws, as states do vary in their reporting laws.)

What if the child's parent/guardian has been traumatized as well?

The concern is that children's trauma may activate their parent's trauma history and limit the positive and supportive ways parents respond to their children. In this situation, parents could benefit from even brief trauma-directed intervention, such as *SITCAP*'s *Adults and Parents in Trauma* program.

What if I have a child whose mother is going through cancer treatments and this sweet first grader is a mess, can I do the program with her now? The standard wait time I know is four to six weeks, but can I do the program with her to help her at this time? If not, what can I do?

Cancer and the process of dying, as well as healing, can be difficult for the entire family as roles and responsibilities change, along with the onset of new worries and anxiety. In this case, this child's mother may no longer be able to care for her child in the same way she did prior to her cancer. Anticipation of the mother's death and so many other possibilities can be frightening and overwhelming for all involved. *SITCAP* would be appropriate as it helps children manage the grief, anxiety, and trauma they can experience as a result of all the changes that can take place as a result of cancer.

I have one boy age 7 who was sexually abused at age 3 by his stepdad, who went to prison and is now out. He has no memory of what bad things his stepdad did, but he

remembers one good thing—that he gave him food to eat. The boy is now acting out sexually with his younger sister. He experiences "good touch and bad touch." What if the "bad touch" feels good?

First, there are many other things we would need to know about this child's history up to his present age, as his behavior may not be related to what he has no memory of happening. A good deal could have happened while his stepfather was in jail. The limited trauma assessment recommended earlier would better determine what matters most to the child.

What if a crisis has just happened in a school? The counselors and social workers need a good reminder of why we wait four to six weeks after the incident to start *SITCAP*. What exactly can they do in the meantime? What are some actual A B C D activities they can initiate?

Chapter 7 presents a detailed response about the reasons we do not initiate *SITCAP* until weeks after initial exposure and which interventions can be most helpful in the first few weeks.

What if I had a client draw a representation of what he felt, not an actual event? It was an adult, and he drew himself in a trash can. At first I thought he meant that this had actually happened to him as a child, but after a few questions I realized it was just how he felt now, thrown away and unwanted. How would I handle this? Would I go with that picture or process that feeling and then ask if he could draw a picture of something he had actually gone through that made him feel that way?

Remaining curious is essential. If this is what he drew, we would pursue it with curiosity and allow his responses to our curiosity to determine where we might go next or what we might ask him to draw next. Only after he has completed the story related to feeling unwanted would we continue with *SITCAP* interventions and the various subjective experiences it addresses.

What if a child is not ready to participate in *SITCAP*; what is my focus?

Much research suggests that the therapeutic relationship between therapist and client is the most important factor leading to positive outcome in therapy (Shirk & Karver, 2003). A therapeutic relationship and environment, built upon trust and positive connection, allows for safety and security (Hawley & Weisz, 2005), both of which are paramount when working with traumatized children and adolescents, whose trust in the adult world has often been violated and shattered.

According to Herman (1992), creating new connections can help resolve trauma by reducing feelings of disconnectedness. The therapeutic relationship helps children recreate a sense of trust, safety, security, and control, in addition to reestablishing healthy boundaries and developing solid attachments (Herman, 1992; Lieberman, Van Horn, &

Ozer, 2005). Children's ability to attach and appropriately interact with others influences how they engage in therapy. Relationship building helps children reestablish trust in the larger community. For many children who experience trauma, the safe and nurturing world they once knew no longer exists. They may lose trust in social systems and individuals whom they once believed would keep them safe. This is why we always return to the importance of making ourselves a safe person to be with while engaging in an intervention that is also deemed safe by the child.

APPENDIX B

SITCAP Program Activity Examples

Each *SITCAP* program has its own manual and workbook containing our sensory-based activities. The manual includes the primary theme of each session, for example, the theme of *worry*. It includes the objectives for each session, the materials needed for that session, the cognitive framing statements presented with each activity for that session, and the steps involved in each activity.

The workbook for each program contains Activity Worksheets referenced by session number and activity number; for example, 1.1 refers to session one, activity one. All worksheets can be copied and used with as many children as participate in *SITCAP*. The worksheets contain a *lined frame*, so the externalization of subjective experiences, sensations, and iconic memories can be contained within that frame. At the top of each worksheet is a brief title of the activity, for example, "This is what happened." Once externalized, we use curiosity and our trauma-specific questioning process to help children bring us further into their world and what matters most.

Given the many different activities covering varying developmental levels and subjective experiences of trauma, we can only include a sampling of worksheets from our different programs in this appendix. For additional information about the programs, go to www.starrtraining.org/tlc or call us at 877-306-5256.

Safety Checklist

Have the child choose how safe/unsafe he feels in the situations below. Younger children can relate to the faces with a simple explanation. "This boy/girl feels safe ... very dangerous.

| 1–Very Safe | 2–Okay | 3–Kind of Dangerous | 4–Very Dangerous |

Rating   **Place**

___ 1.	My bedroom
___ 2.	My house
___ 3.	My neighborhood
___ 4.	The nearest park
___ 5.	My school (overall)
___ 6.	The halls at school
___ 7.	The gym
___ 8.	My bus stop*
___ 9.	The bathrooms at school
___ 10.	The bus I take to school*
___ 11.	The cafeteria
___ 12.	The way home from school
___ 13.	At my locker
___ 14.	In my classrooms
___ 15.	At the movies
___ 16.	While riding my bike
___ 17.	At the mall or the local stores
___ 18.	With my father
___ 19.	With my mother
___ 20.	With my brother(s) or sister(s)*
___ 21.	With my extended family (aunts, uncles, cousins, etc.)
___ 22.	With my friends
___ 23.	At parties or social gathering

Structured Sensory Interventions for Traumatized Children, Adolescents and Parents: At-Risk Adjudicated Residential Treatment Program

Worksheet 3.2a – This is Me

This is me:

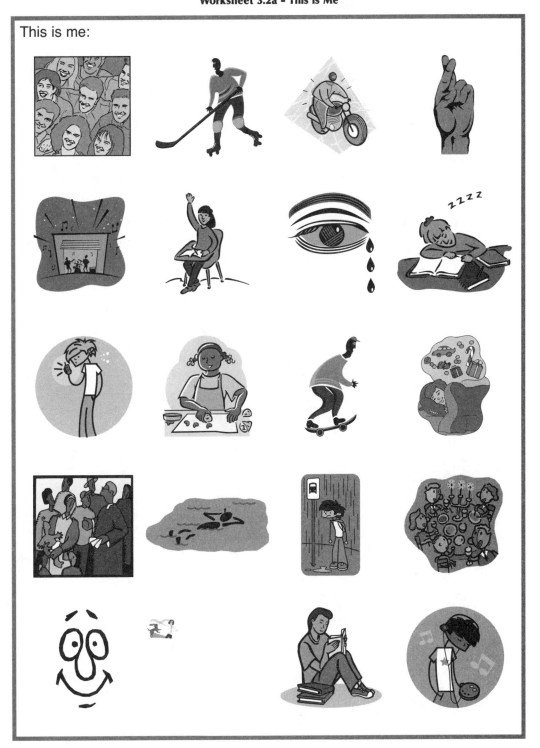

Structured Sensory Interventions for Traumatized Children, Adolescents and Parents: At-Risk Adjudicated Residential Treatment Program
Worksheet 3.2b – This is Me

This is me:

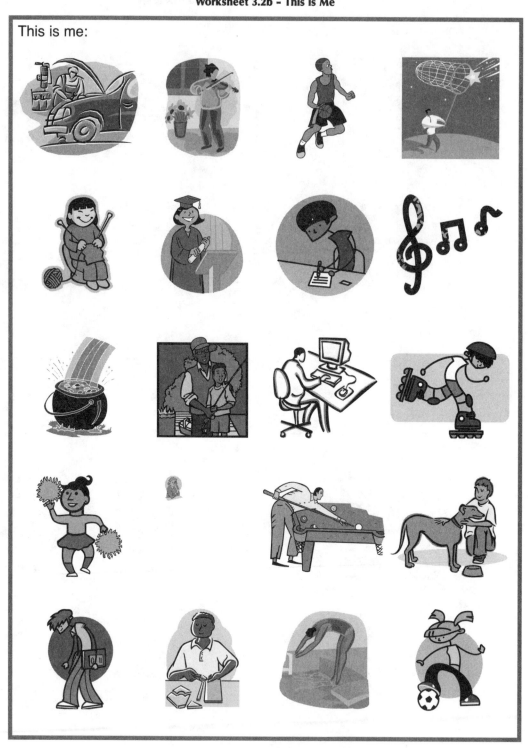

Structured Sensory Interventions for Traumatized Children, Adolescents and Parents: At-Risk Adjudicated Residential Treatment Program

Worksheet 3.2c – This is Me

This is me:

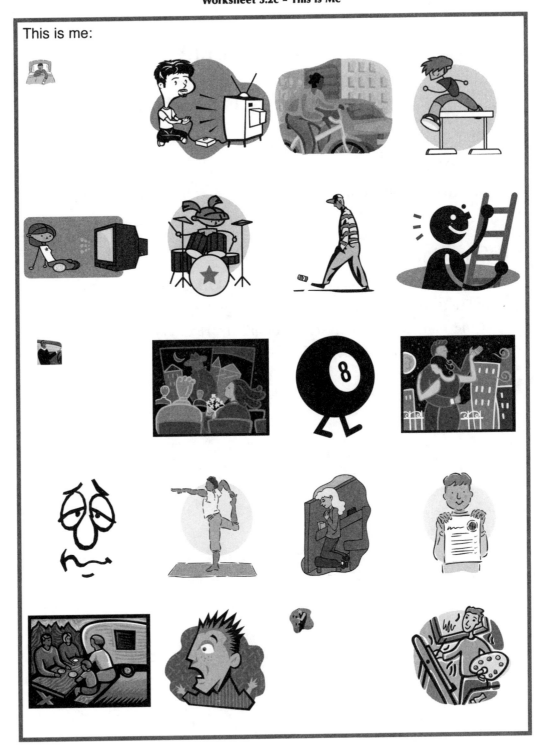

One-Minute Interventions for Traumatized Children and Adolescents
Ages 3-5

WORRY

My Worry is as Big As . . .

Directions:

Ask the child to color in the image that represents how big their worry is.

Reframing:

When it rains it doesn't rain forever, does it? NO. Worries don't last forever either. Some worries seem like there is nothing we can do to change them or stop them. But we can't do anything to stop the rain either, but it stops doesn't it? YES. And when it rains don't we usually find something to do until it stops? Sure we do.

One-Minute Interventions for Traumatized Children and Adolescents
Ages 3–5

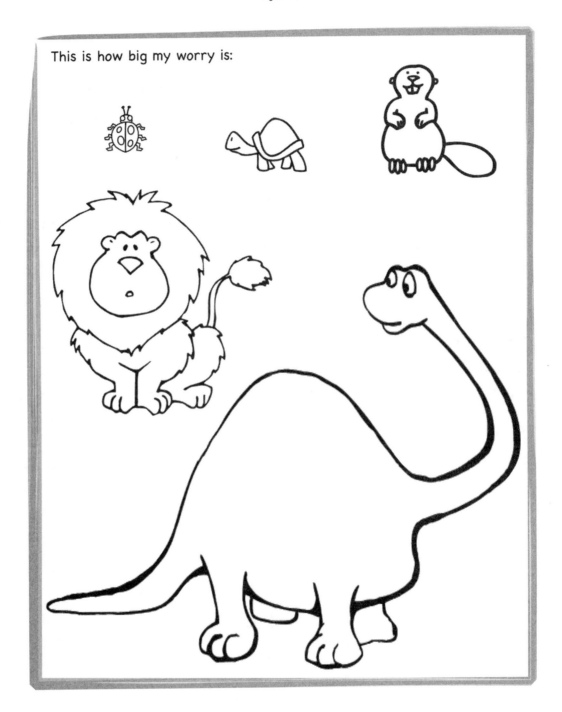

This is how big my worry is:

One-Minute Interventions for Traumatized Children and Adolescents
Ages 13-18

ANGER

If I Could Say One or Two Words
That Would Explain How Mad I was, I Would Say . . .

Directions:

Ask the adolescent to list one or two words that best explain how they feel or what they'd like to say when they are really mad. Have the youngster write those words really big on the paper and color them in if they wish. Then allow the youngster to say, scream, or yell those one or two words very loudly several times in your office.

Reframing:

Sometimes when we get really mad it helps us just to yell really loud, scream out a word or two that expresses how we feel. We often don't need anyone to hear us; we just have to get it out. The next time you are really mad, go into your basement, your bedroom, or outside and yell or scream out those one or two words that help let you express your anger.

One-Minute Interventions for Traumatized Children and Adolescents
Ages 13-18

If I could say one or two words that would explain how mad I was,
I would say...

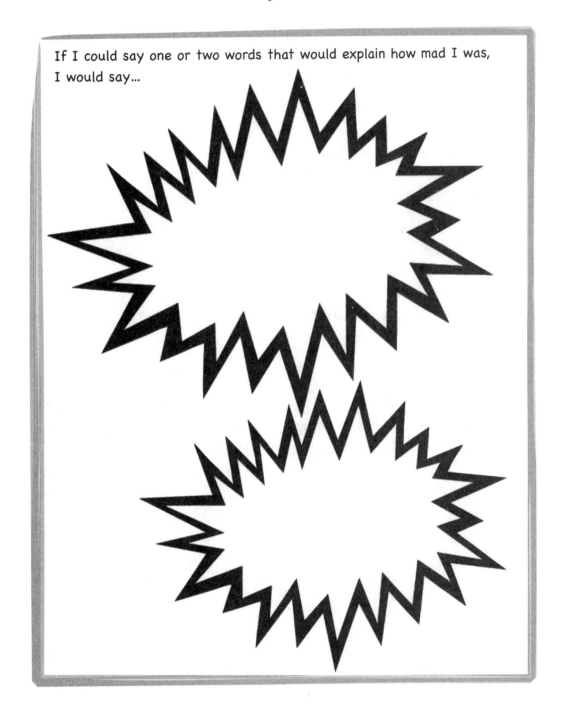

Helping Children Feel Safe 57
(This activity developed by Nancy C. Klein)

BUBBLE CIRCUS

Age range: Kindergarten through fourth grade

Materials:

➡ Drawing paper, crayons (optional: bubbles)
➡ Optional read-aloud book: *Bedtime for Frances* by R. Hoben.
➡ Bubble Circus Activity Sheet #16

Theme: Distressful thoughts may make it difficult to fall asleep. It is helpful to focus on pleasant images in order to put distressful thoughts in the background.

When we are worried, our minds are filled with questions and concerns. It may be difficult to clear our heads and relax so that we can fall asleep. Do you have a special routine that helps you feel calm and sleepy? What are some books that are good to read before bedtime?

Possible areas of concern:

"I don't want to go to bed because when I do I feel lonely and I get sad." "I'm afraid to fall asleep because I have bad dreams." Other people have these troubles, too. It's good to have a few different ideas that you can use if you ever have trouble falling asleep. What are some ideas that might help you clear your mind and feel relaxed? (Responses may include drinking a warm cup of milk, listening to soft music, having a night-light, looking at a comforting picture, holding a cuddly object, saying special things.) Be sure not to watch scary shows or read scary stories before you go to bed.

Activity:

A really good way to fall asleep is to think calm, happy thoughts. (Suggest that he/she may wish to try this with you.)

Imagine that you have a bottle of bubbles in your hand. Pretend to make a large bubble and watch it float above you. Picture a funny animal inside your bubble. The animal is doing circus tricks for you. Blow more imaginary bubbles and pretend that you have a whole circus of bubbles to watch. This makes you feel relaxed and happy. When the circus show is over you will be ready to fall asleep.

Activity Extension:

(If you have a bottle of bubbles available, begin the drawing activity by blowing some bubbles.) Suggest that the child draw a picture of a favorite activity. They may wish to draw the imaginary bubble circus. Let the child take the picture home and use it as a reminder to think about pleasant things before falling asleep.

Helping Children Feel Safe
Bubble Circus Extension Activity Sheet #16

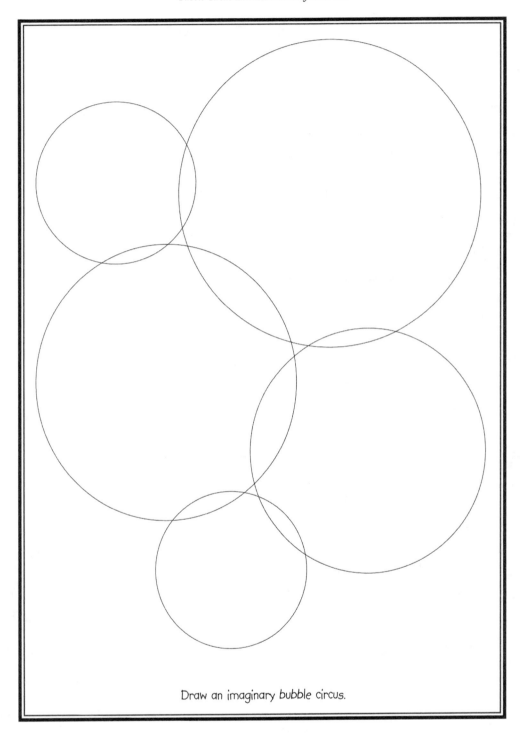

Draw an imaginary bubble circus.

Secondary Wounding

Has anyone said to you . . .

If anyone, including doctors, nurses, police officers, social workers, clergy, or others said any of the following, you have been further victimized. This may be hard to believe because the comments have come from people you expected help and support you.

Which of the following comments have been said to you?

_____

_____You are exaggerating!

_____It couldn't have happened that way.

_____You really can't remember that kind of detail.

_____Your imagination is running away with you.

_____He/she would never do that.

_____There are people who have had it harder than you.

_____Consider yourself lucky.

_____You're still young.

_____You're overreacting. You need to put this in perspective.

_____What happened, happened. You don't need to be upset.

_____Well maybe if you hadn't. . . .

_____Well maybe if you had. . . .

_____If only you. . . .

_____You should have never . . .

_____That wasn't very smart of you.

_____How many times have you been told. . . .

_____It wouldn't have happened if you. . . .

_____You must have wanted for it to have happened.

_____You must have been looking for trouble.

_____You need to be more careful.

If any one of these statements have been made to you, you have been wounded. A person's "wounding" can be as difficult to recover from as multiple wounds. Betrayal is betrayal, whether it happened once or twice. If you did have multiple, secondary victimization there is a greater likelihood that you also experience a high level of guilt and self-blame, which is keeping you thinking as a "victim."

Other remarks _____

School Recovery Protocol

TLC's recommended recovery protocols are derived from 23 years of assisting schools following critical incidents. They support the primary components of trauma-informed practices and trauma-informed care. As in all *SITCAP* programs, our recovery protocols are also contained in a manual titled *Traumatic Event Crisis Incident Planning (TECIP)*. TLC publishes *TECIP*, which combines TLC-recommended recovery protocol and those developed by the staff of Copes Consulting, a school-based staff that is experienced in recovery protocol. Several of the examples included in this appendix were referenced in Chapter 7. For further information about *TECIP*, please visit us at www.starrtraining. org/tlc or call us at 877-306-5256.

Fan Out Meeting Agenda/Traumatic Event Briefing

First (Fan Out) Staff Meeting

The meeting with staff to inform them of the incident and prepare them for student response needs to present the following messages:

1. Factual data related to death. Warning: If method of death is questionable, students, parents, etc. are to be told only that the manner of death is still under investigation by the coroner's office.

2. Rumors about the incident are to be reported immediately to the Trauma Team. (Identify a specific person if possible.)

3. This is a time when many students may discharge a residue of emotion which has nothing to do with the deceased, but provides them with an acceptable vehicle for catharsis. Any concerns about student emotional stability and risk is to be directed to the team immediately for assessment.

4. How to "transport" upset students to the Trauma Team or how to bring the Team to the student(s) if necessary.

5. All media questions etc. are to be directed to the assigned Administrator (i.e., principal, superintendent).

6. Staff will be informed of any new information that is provided to the Administration.

7. Staff are expected to meet again after school to debrief what took place during the day.

8. Staff need to hear that no one can predict what kinds of reactions they may see in students, staff, or even themselves and that at the after-school meeting possible reactions will be further addressed.

9. The announcement to be read or presented to students must be reviewed and teachers given some guidance as to responding to student reactions such as:

   a. Students having a difficult time can be seen by the Trauma Team

   b. Students can be assured they will have an opportunity as a group to hear and talk more

   c. Let students ask questions; note those questions the teacher cannot answer so that they can be addressed in the classroom presentation or as new information becomes available

   d. It is okay for them, as teachers, to express their shock, sadness, tears, or difficulty with talking about the deceased and that they, too, are looking forward to the classroom presentation

10. Staff need reassurance that there is enough staff support available (i.e., substitute teachers, team members from other schools, etc. should the response demand additional support). It is advisable that one or two trained people be identified as available during the day for staff people to talk with about their own reactions and concerns if needed.

Classroom Presentation Guide
Developed by TLC

The purpose of a classroom presentation activity is to provide information, minimize unwanted student responses, normalize grief and trauma reactions, and suggest appropriate behavior. Five primary steps guide this process.

1. **Introduce discussion**

   As some of you may already know, _____. This is very difficult for all of us. When something like this happens, it is hard to know what to say or how to act. It is important, however, that we spend some time talking about this incident and answer any questions that you might have.

2. **Clarify the facts**

   This is what we know so far _____. We do not know anything else. As we find out more information that you need to know, we will share it with you (may want to emphasize the importance of not starting rumors—see #4).

3. **Normalize common reactions**

   What did you think and feel when you first heard about this? What are you thinking and feeling now? I am not surprised that you feel this way, or have these kind of thoughts. Sometimes I feel and think this way. These are very normal reactions. If they are really bothering you, it usually helps to talk to someone about what you are thinking and feeling.

4. **Identify appropriate behavior**

   When you have felt upset in the past, what kinds of things have you done to help you feel better? What have you seen other people do to help them? Here are some things that I have seen other people do _____. Sometimes people begin to spread rumors. This is not helpful to the family or close friends. If you hear anything different from what we have talked about, please let us know and we will check it out.

5. **Conclude discussion**

   Are there any questions before we end? If at any time during the next several days you want to talk to someone, please let a teacher know. For the remainder of the period I would like for us to _____ (consider adjusting activity depending on student response). Inform students of building resources that are available and tell them that they will be informed of new information.

Traumatic Event Crisis Intervention Plan
Student Re-Entry Plan
(Published by TLC)

Consider the following best practice strategies and accommodations for a student who is returning to the school after a significant event. These are students who are considered "closest to the trauma."

Prior to Student Return: A Modified Classroom Discussion

The classroom(s) that the student in question attends should consider having a brief discussion prior to re-entry. But what should be discussed? Here are some suggested talking points to consider.

➤ "Good morning class, I want to take a moment to talk about (name of student). As we discussed, (name of student) has (suffered a great loss/recently been through a very difficult time). I'm glad to report that (name of student) will be returning to class on _____ and I think we should take a moment to talk about some things we can do or not do to make his/her return to school as positive a possible."

➤ "First and foremost, like any other day here at school, we need to show respect for one another. In being respectful to _____, please don't bombard _____ with questions about what has happened. If he/she wants to talk about it, that will be his/her choice to do so."

➤ "Remind yourself what it means to be a friend to someone. How do you want to be treated by others? It's perfectly normal to want to be there for a friend in need. If you have the urge to tell ____ that you are sorry about what happened, that's ok. That's a nice gesture. It's ok to share with ____ that if he/she wants to talk that you'll be there for him/her."

➤ "It's also ok if you don't know what to say to ____. When something like this happens, we may feel unsure of what the right words are to say to someone. Again, this is normal. To say nothing is ok too."

➤ "Remember, our class is a safe place to be and we want nothing more than to have everyone here feel that they are safe and that they belong."

➤ "The best thing you can do is to treat _____ with the respect he/she deserves, just as you do."

➤ If you have questions, concerns, or see someone treating ____ in a way you feel is inappropriate, let a staff member know so they can intervene/ help."

The Day the Student Returns: Working with the Returning Student

Morning of the return:
It is suggested that upon returning to the school, a brief meeting is held with the student (possibly accompanied by their guardian) to let the student be reassured that they are an important person in the school, that the school is a safe place to be, and that support is available to them should they feel the need.

Being mindful that the student has the right to choose how they cope with the event and their emotional reactions to the event, the school should share several options/accommodations for the student. Some students may not use any of the suggested accommodations because they don't want to feel like they are getting "special treatment." Nonetheless, the opportunity for the student to have such supports available is certainly recommended.

> *Having several key people who the student has a rapport with be "on-call" that first week back should the student be in need of having to talk to someone.*
> *Having a location nearby the student's classroom where he/she can go to "regroup" either by his/herself or with a classmate of their choosing.*
> *Have the guardian on-call should emotional reactions be too overwhelming that first or second day back to school.*
> *Consider a modified schedule if the transition appears to be "too much too soon" – possibly go to half days for the first week back if necessary.*
> *Provide added support in less structured settings (i.e., lunch room, recess). If this is not possible, make sure staff assigned to these areas are updated regarding the return of the student and to be aware of any activity in these settings that may be hurtful to the student.*

Midday Update:
It may be advisable to have an identified key person check in on the student to see how the day is progressing for them.

> Does the student have any concerns or questions?
> Do they want to call their guardian just to let them know that how they are doing?
> Remind the student of the options discussed and ask if they felt the need to utilize any accommodations so far.

*If you feel that having morning, midday, and end-of-the-day meetings is too overwhelming and unnecessary, don't have the meeting. It is important to use your judgment in determining the need.

End of Day:
As the end of the day approaches, it may be advisable to have a final, albeit brief, update meeting to see how the day's return went from the perspective of the student. An activity to gauge how their day went is provided below.

Ask the student the following:

> *"On a scale of 1-10; 1 being that the day was very overwhelming and very difficult and 10 being that the day was very positive, where would you rank how the day went?*

The response could help determine an action plan for subsequent days. A response of 4 or lower may mean that another meeting is warranted to determine what appropriate course of action should be taken.

A response of 5 or greater may mean that the supports for the following day may remain in place. Ask the student if they would be willing to have another meeting at the end of the next day to see if there has been any progress.

Ask the student what measure might be taken to help them move up 1 or 2 numbers on that scale.

Modify the day two plan accordingly based on the responses.

Resilience Resources for Teachers

As discussed in our final chapter, resiliency is learned. The school classroom and school environments provide multiple opportunities for children to develop resilience, when taught by their teachers and supported by school policies and practices. Resilient children are better able to regulate their behaviors and are generally more effective learners than are nonresilient children. It only makes sense that the adults who spend five days a week with children at school also be involved in presenting them with lessons leading to resilience. The resources presented in this appendix provide many specific activities that teachers can incorporate into their classrooms and teaching methods.

Resources for Resilience in Schools

Resilience Net is the best provider of international, current information and research about resilience. This site contains bibliographies, links to other resilience websites, and tips on resilience promotion. This site is for researchers, professionals, parents, and youth. www.resilnet.uiuc.edu

Tribes provides information on transforming schools into positive learning communities. Tribes's mission is to ensure the healthy development of every child so that each has the knowledge, competency, and resilience to be successful. www.tribes.com

The National Network for Family Resiliency: http://www.nnfr.org

The Search Institute website focuses on the 40 assets that all young people need. http://search-institute.org

The Tucson Resiliency Initiative site contains strategies for building resilient youth, best practices, and success stories. www.tucsonresiliency.org

Thrivenet is a resource website for learning about resilience, thriving, and how to gain strength from adversity. www.thrivenet.com

Resiliency in Action strives to spread resiliency news, including research, applications, and evaluation of resilience programs. www.resiliency.com

Project Resilience website for resiliency researchers includes training and a project guide, links, and a discussion group. Description and links to scientifically proven programs for violence prevention, including those that build resiliency. www.projectresilience.com

Recognizing Youth as Resources empowers youth to positively affect their communities through civic involvement. www.ryar.org

About the Authors

William Steele, PsyD, MSW, MA, founded the National Institute for Trauma and Loss in Children (TLC) in 1990 after 20 years of assisting children and families in crisis. In the early to mid-1980s, he traveled the country assisting schools and clinics with developing their responses to the epidemic of suicide among young people, and in the late 1980s, he helped with their responses to the emergence of violence as an epidemic taking the lives of young children and adolescents. Dr. Steele has assisted survivors following such tragedies as the Gulf War; the bombing of the Federal Building in Oklahoma; 9/11 in New York, Washington, D.C., and Virginia; Hurricanes Katrina and Rita; numerous acts of deadly violence in school settings; and the day-to-day traumatizing of children that rarely receives national media attention. His most recent publication, *Trauma-Informed Practices with Children and Adolescents*, speaks to his experience and knowledge in the field of trauma. He developed *Structured Sensory Interventions for Traumatized Children, Adolescents and Parents (SITCAP®)*, a series of intervention programs that is registered on the California Clearinghouse of Evidence-Based Practices and the Substance Abuse Mental Health Services Agency's registry of evidence-based practices.

Dr. Steele has trained more than 60,000 professionals and has had numerous publications in such journals and periodicals as the *School Social Work Journal*, *Residential Treatment for Children and Youth*, *National Social Sciences*, *Reclaiming Children and Youth*, *Child and Family Professional*, and *USA Today*. He has also contributed numerous chapters about working with traumatized children for such publications as *Understanding Mass Violence*, *Handbook of Art Therapy*, and *Critical Incidents in Counseling Children*, and he is a published author with Learning Publications, Guilford Press, and Routledge.

Dr. Steele founded TLC to advance and make available trauma-informed practices for children and adolescents. Today there are 6,000 TLC Certified Trauma Specialists he has personally trained, and they are now practicing TLC's evidence-based interventions worldwide. When asked, he will tell you that he is most proud of the thousands of practitioners who have volunteered so much of their time to field test, research, and help develop TLC's intervention programs. Since the founding of TLC, Dr. Steele has insisted that interventions not direct themselves to treating symptoms, which can be misleading, but to first discovering the way children are actually experiencing themselves, us, and their worlds as a result of their exposure to overwhelming and terrifying situations. For years he has provided practitioners with the training, interventions, and resources needed to be able to see what traumatized children see when they look at themselves and their world, as a way to discover what matters most in their efforts to heal and flourish. Today TLC is a program of the Starr Global Learning Network of Starr Commonwealth, which has been creating environments where children flourish for more than 100 years.

Caelan Kuban, PsyD, LMSW, is Director of the National Institute for Trauma and Loss in Children (TLC), a program of the Starr Global Learning Network. Dr. Kuban provides training across the country to professionals working with traumatized children and families and has been called an excellent teacher and passionate trainer, providing workshops where participants leave feeling energized and inspired to work with at-risk and traumatized youth. Participants have written, "This is the best presentation I have attended in 20 years" and "She has a way of making difficult content easy to grasp." As TLC's Director, Dr. Kuban has successfully brought together agency-wide trauma certification trainings across the country with such organizations as the Virtual Center of Excellence and Wayne County Community Mental Health in Michigan, Ohio Association of Child Care Agencies, the Circle of Hope in Missouri, and a 17-county, trauma-informed initiative in North Carolina. Dr. Kuban has coordinated and completed several evidence-based research studies, including *Children of Today* with at-risk, 6- to 12-year-old school-aged children in Michigan and *Restoring Hope and Resiliency* with at-risk and adjudicated adolescents in Ohio and Georgia. Both studies showed outstanding, statistically significant results across trauma subscales and mental health categories.

She is the author of the TLC publications *Zero to Three: A Handbook of Trauma Interventions, One-Minute Trauma Interventions, More One-Minute Trauma Interventions*, and *A Time for Resilience*, in addition to numerous articles, in such journals as the *School Social Work Journal, Children and Schools, Residential Treatment for Children and Youth, Reclaiming Children and Youth*, and *Child Family Professional*, and she is a contributor to *Mental Health Issues of Child Maltreatment*. Dr. Kuban also coordinated the development of 30 TLC online courses approved by all major providers of continuing education and, while continuing her administrative duties, provides ongoing supervision with TLC Certified Trauma Specialists.

References

ACFASP Scientific Review. (2010). Critical Incident Stress Debriefing (CISD). Retrieved May 11, 2012, from www.instructorscorner.org/media/resources/SAC/Reviews/Critical%20%20Stress%20CISD

Achenbach, T. M., & Rescorla, L. A. (2001). *Manual for the ASEBA school-age: Forms & profiles*. Burlington: University of Vermont, Research Center for Children, Youth, & Families.

Adler, A. (1930). *The problem child.* New York, NY: P. G. Putnam's Sons.

Alisic, E., Boeije, H. R., Jongmans, M. J., & Kleber, R. J. (2011). Children's perspectives on dealing with traumatic events. Journal of Loss and Trauma, 16, 477–496.

Alisic, E., van der Schoot, T. A., van Ginkel, J. R., & Kleber, R. J. (2008). Looking beyond posttraumatic stress stress disorder in children: Posttraumatic stress reactions, posttraumatic growth and quality of life in general population sample. *Journal of Clinical Psychiatry, 69,* 1455–1461.

Allan, J. (1988). *Inscapes of the child's world: Jungian counseling in schools and clinics.* Dallas, TX: Spring Publications.

American Psychological Association (APA). (1980). *Diagnostic and statistical manual of mental disorders* (3rd ed. rev., DSM-III-R). Washington, DC: Author.

American Psychological Association (APA). (1994). *Diagnostic and statistical manual of mental disorders* (4th ed., DSM-IV). Washington, DC: Author.

American Psychological Association (APA). (2000). *Diagnostic and statistical manual of mental disorders* (text rev., DSM-IV-TR). Washington, DC: Author.

American Psychological Association (APA). (2012). DSM-5 development. Retrieved October 25, 2012, from www.dsm5.org/ProposedRevisions/Pages/proposedrevision.aspx?rid=165

American Psychological Association, Presidential Task Force on Evidence-Based Practice. (2005, August). *Policy statement on evidence-based practice.* Retrieved June 18, 2007, from www2.apa.org/practice/ebstatement.pdf

Atwool, N. (2006). Attachment and resilience: Implications for children in care. *Child Care in Practice, 12*(4), 315–330.

Azar, B. (2011). Oxytocin's other side. *American Psychological Association, 42*(3), 40.

Bath, H. (2008). The three pillars of trauma-informed care. *Reclaiming Children and Youth, 17*(3), 5.

Berberian, M., Bryant L., & Landsburg, M. (2003). Interventions with communities affected by mass violence. In C. Malchiodi (Ed.), *Handbook of art therapy*. New York, NY: Guilford Press.

Betancourt, T. S., & Khan, K. T. (2008). The mental health of children affected by armed conflict: Protective processes and pathways to resilience. *International Review of Psychiatry, 20*(3), 317–328.

Beuchler, S. (2004). *Clinical values and emotions that guide psychoanalytical treatment*. New York, NY: Taylor & Francis.

Beyers, J. (1996). Children of the stones: Art therapy interventions in the West Bank. *Art Therapy: Journal of the American Art Therapy Association, 13*, 238–243.

Bickart, T., & Wolin, S. (1997). Practicing resilience in elementary classrooms. Retrieved February 14, 2012, from www.projectresilience.com/article17.htm

Bloom, S. L., & Farragher, B. (2010). *Destroying sanctuary: The crisis in human service delivery systems*. New York, NY: Oxford University Press.

Bolin, I. (2010). Chillihuani's culture of respect and the Circle of Courage. *Reclaiming Children and Youth, 18*(4), 12–17.

Bonanno, G. A., Wortman, C. B., Lehman, D. R., Tweed, R. G., Haring, M., Sonnega, J., . . . Nesse, R. M. (2002). Resilience to loss and chronic grief: A prospective study from pre-loss to 18-months post-loss. *Journal of Personality and Social Psychology, 83*, 1150–1164.

Bonanno, G. A., Wortman, C. B., & Nesse, R. M. (2004). Prospective patterns of resilience and maladjustment during widowhood. *Psychology and Aging, 19*, 260–271.

Bowlby, J., & Winton, J. (1998). *Attachment and loss: Separation, anger and anxiety*. New York, NY: Basic Books.

Bremner, J. D. (2001). A biological model of delayed recall of childhood abuse. *Journal of Aggression, Maltreatment and Trauma, 4*, 165–183.

Bremner, J. D., Krystal, J. H., Charnez, D. S., & Southwick, S. M. (1996). Neural mechanisms in dissociative amnesia for childhood abuse: Relevance to the current controversy surrounding the false memory syndrome. *American Journal of Psychiatry, 153*(7), 71–80.

Brendtro, L., Brokenleg, M., & Van Bockern, S. (2002). *Reclaiming youth at risk: Our hope for the future*. Indianapolis, IN: Solution Tree.

Brendtro, L., & Longhurst, J. (2005). The resilient brain. *Reclaiming Children and Youth, 14*(1), 52–60.

Brendtro, L., Mitchell, M., & McCall, H. (2009). *Deep brain learning: Pathways to potential with challenging youth*. Albion, MI: Starr Commonwealth.

Brent, D., Perper, J., Moritz, G., Friend, A., Schweers, J., Allman, C., . . . Balach, L. (1993). Adolescent witnesses to peer suicide. *Journal of the American Academy of Child and Adolescent Psychiatry, 32*(6), 1184–1188.

Briere, J. (1996). *Trauma symptom checklist for children*. Odessa, FL: Psychological Assessment Resources.

Brokenleg, M. (2012). Humanized youth work. *Reclaiming Children and Youth, 20*(4), 10–12.

Bronfenbrenner, U. (Ed.). (2005). *Making human beings human: Bioecological perspectives on human development*. Thousand Oaks, CA: Sage.

Brooks, R. B., & Goldstein, S. (2012). 10 ways to make your child more resilient. Retrieved November 11, 2012, from www.familytlc.net/resilient_children_preteen.html

Bryk, A., & Schneider, B. (2002). *Trust in schools: A core resource for improvement.* New York, NY: Russell Sage Foundation.

Buechler, S. (2004). *Clinical values: Emotions that guide psychoanalytic treatment.* Hillsdale, NJ: Analytic Press.

Burnham, J. J. (2009). Contemporary fears of children and adolescents: Coping and resiliency in the 21st century. *Journal of Counseling & Development, 87*(1), 28–35.

Cahn, B. R., & Polich, J. (2006). Meditation states and traits: EEG, ERP and neuro-imaging studies. *Psychological Bulletin, 132*(2), 180.

Calhoun, L. G., & Tedeschi, R. G. (2006). *The assessment of posttraumatic growth in different cultural contexts.* Symposium presented at the annual meeting of the International Society for Traumatic Stress Studies, Hollywood, California.

Carlton, G., Markowitz, M., Hadow, J., & Steele, W. (2011). *After the crisis: Traumatic Event Crisis Intervention Plan (TECIP).* Clinton Township, MI: TLC Institute.

Catalano, R. F., & Hawkins, J. D. (1996). The social development model: A theory of antisocial behavior. In J. D. Hawkins (Ed)., *Delinquency and crime: Current theories* (pp. 149–197). New York, NY: Cambridge University Press.

Centers for Disease Control and Prevention (CDC). (2011). Adverse child experiences (ACE) study. Retrieved March 30, 2011, from www.cdc.gov/ace/index.htm

Chen, Jie-Qi, Moran, S., & Gardner, H. (2009). *Multiple intelligences around the world.* New York, NY: Jossey-Bass.

Coifman, K. G., Bonnano, G. A., Ray, R. D., & Gross J. J. (2007). Does repressive coping promote resilience? Affective-autonomic response discrepancy during bereavement. *Journal of Personality and Social Psychology, 92*(4), 745–758.

Cloitre, M., Morin, N., & Linares, L. O. (2004). *Children's resilience in the face of trauma.* New York: New York University Child Study Center.

Cloud, J. (2010, January). Why your DNA isn't your destiny. Retrieved January 15, 2012, from www.time.com/time/health/articles/0,8599,1951968,00.html

Collins, D. (2009). *Essentials of business ethics: Creating an organization of high integrity and superior performance.* Hoboken, NJ: Wiley.

Condy, A., & Kehman, P. (2007). *Theoretical perspectives for direct social work practice.* Google eBook.

Connors, R., & Smith, T. (2009). *How did that happen? Holding people accountable for results the positive principled way.* New York, NY: Penguin.

Copeland, W. E., Anglod, K. G., & Costello, E. J. (2007). Traumatic events and posttraumatic stress in childhood. *Archives of General Psychiatry, 64,* 577–584.

Dallman-Jones, A. (2006). *Shadow children: Understanding education's #1 problem.* Lancaster, PA: RLD Publications.

Davis, K. M. (2010). Music and expressive arts with children experiencing trauma. *Journal of Creativity in Mental Health, 5*(2), 125–133.

Dietrich, R. (2008). Evidence-based education: Can we get there from here? *Association for Behavioral Analysis International, 31*(3). Retrieved December 12, 2012, from www.abainternational.org/ABA/newsletter/vol313/Detrich.asp

Divorce and PTSD. (2012). Retrieved February 14, 2012 from www.divorce.com/article/divorce-ptsd

Echterling, L. G., Presbury, J. H., & McKee, J. E. (2005). *Crisis intervention: Promoting resilience and resolution in troubled times.* Upper Saddle River, NJ: Prentice Hall.

Emerson, D., Hopper, E., van der Kolk, B., & Levine, P. (2011). *Overcoming trauma through yoga: Reclaiming your body.* Berkeley, CA: North Atlantic Books.

Filipovic, Z. (1999). *The freedom writers diary: How a teacher and 150 teens used writing to change themselves and the world around them.* New York, NY: Doubleday.

Fischer, K. (2012). Neuroscience in the classroom: Making connections, section 2. Retrieved June 5, 2012, from www.Learner.org/neuroscience/text.html?dis=u&num=05&Sec=02

Fishbane, M. (2007). Wired to connect: Neuroscience, relationships, and therapy. *Family Process, 46*(3), 395–412.

Fletcher, K. E. (2003). Childhood posttraumatic stress disorder. In E. J. Marsh & R. A. Barkley (Eds.), *Child psychopathology* (2nd ed., pp. 310–371). New York, NY: Guilford Press.

Foa, E. B., Keane, T. M., Friedman, M. J., & Cohen, J. A. (2008). *Effective treatments for PTSD: Practice guidelines from the International Society for Traumatic Stress Studies.* New York, NY: Guilford Press.

Ford, J., Chapman, J., Mack, M., & Pearson, G. (2006). Pathways from traumatic child victimization to delinquency: Implications for juvenile permanency court proceedings and decisions. *Juvenile and Family Court Journal, Winter,* 13–26.

Fosha, D. (2000). *The transformation power of affect: A model of accelerated change.* New York, NY: Baha Books.

Freado, M. (2010). Measuring the impact of Re-ED. *Reclaiming Children and Youth, 19*(2), 28–31.

Gao, T. (2008). Music therapy and crisis intervention with survivors of the China earthquake of May 12, 2008. Retrieved February 15, 2011, from www.chinamusictherapy.org/html/data/en/a38.html

Gharabaghi, K. (2008). Reclaiming our "toughest" youth. *Reclaiming Children and Youth, 17*(3), 30–32.

Gil, E. (2003). Art and play therapy with sexually abused children. In C. Malchiodi (Ed.), *Handbook of art therapy* (pp. 152–166). New York, NY: Guilford Press.

Gil, E. (2006). *Helping abused and traumatized children: Integrating directive and nondirective approaches.* New York, NY: Guilford Press.

Ginsburg, K. R. (2006). *Building resilience in children and teens: Giving kids roots and wings.* Washington, DC: American Academy of Pediatrics.

Golub, D. (1985). Symbolic expression in post traumatic stress disorder: Vietnam combat veterans in art therapy. *The Arts in Psychotherapy, 12,* 285–296.

Goodin, J., & Abernathy, J. (2011). Press release from the American Academy of Orthopedic Surgeons regarding PTSD. Retrieved February 6, 2012, from www.indianapolisinjury.net/blog/detail/press-release-from-the-american-academy-orthopedic-surgeons-ptsd

Gratz, K. L., & Roemer, L. (2004). Multidimensional assessment of motional regulation and dysregulation: Development, factor, structure and initial validation of the Difficulties in Emotional Regulation Scale. *Journal of Psychopathology and Behavioral Assessment, 36,* 41–54.

Green, J. A., Whitney, P. G., & Potegal, M. (2011). Screaming, yelling, whining, and crying: Categorical and intensity differences in vocal expressions of anger and sadness in children's tantrums. *Emotion, 11*(5), 1124–1133.

Gross, J., & Haynes, H. (1998). Drawing facilitates children's verbal reports of emotionally laden events. *Journal of Experimental Psychology, 4*, 163–179.

Hawley, K. M., & Weisz, J. R. (2005). Youth versus parent working alliance in usual clinical care: Distinctive associations with retention, satisfaction and treatment outcome. *Journal of Clinical Child and Adolescent Psychology, 34*, 117–128.

Heller, L., & Lapierre, A. (2012). *How early developmental trauma affects self regulation, self image & the capacity for relationship.* Berkeley, CA: North Atlantic Books.

Henrikson, B. (2012). The present moment: A gateway to resilience. Retrieved May 5, 2012, from www.livingwellfeelinggood.com/2012/01

Henry, J. (2011). Stuffed animals may ease war-related stress in kids. Retrieved June 4, 2012, from www.reuters.com/article/2008/01/11/us-stuffed-kids-idUSHAR16990320080111

Herman, J. L. (1992). *Trauma and recovery.* New York, NY: Basic Books.

Hill, C., & Updegraff, J. (2012). Mindfulness and its relationship to emotional regulation. *Emotion, 12*(1), 81–90.

Hodas, G. (2006). Responding to childhood trauma. Retrieved January 15, 2012, from www.nasmhpd.org/general_files/publications/ntac_pubs/RespondingtoChildhoodTrauma-Hodas.pdf

Hoover-Dempsey, K. V., Batitiato, A. C., Walker, J. M. T., Reed, R. P., DeJong, J. M., & Jones, K. P. (2001). Parental involvement in homework. *Educational Psychologist, 36*(3), 195–209.

Hoven, C., Durate, C., Lucas, C. P., Wu, P., Mandell, D. J., Goodwin, R. D., . . . Susser, E. (2005). Psychopathology among New York City public school children 6 months after September 11. *Archives of General Psychiatry, 62*, 545–552.

Hughes, R. (2009). Attachment-focused treatment for children. In M. Kerman (Ed.), *Clinical pearls of wisdom* (pp. 169–181). New York, NY: W. W. Norton.

Hurd, N., & Zimmerman, M. (2010). Natural mentoring relationships among adolescent mothers: A study of resilience. *Journal of Research on Adolescents, 20*, 789–809.

Hyman, I. A., & Snook, P. A. (1999). *Dangerous schools: What we can do about the physical and emotional abuse of our children.* San Francisco, CA: Jossey-Bass.

Jeang Lee, S. (2007). The relations between the student–teacher trust relationship and school success in the case of Korean middle schools. *Educational Studies, 33*(2), 209–216.

Jewett-Jarett, C. (2000). *Helping children cope with separation and loss.* Boston, MA: The Harvard Common Press.

Kahneman, D. (2011). Daniel Kahneman: The riddle of experience vs. memory. Video. Retrieved November 17, 2012, from www.ted.com/. . ./daniel_kahneman_the_riddle_of_experience_vs_me

Kasdin, A. E. (2000). *Psychotherapy for children and adolescents: Directions for research and practice.* New York, NY: Oxford University Press.

Kashdan, T. (2011). Post-traumatic distress and the presence of post-traumatic growth and meaning in life: Experiential avoidance as a moderator. Retrieved January 12, 2012, from www.Elsevier-com/personality-and-individual-differences/#

Kates, A. (2009). *PTSD can attack years later: Even with no previous symptoms*. Retrieved February 16, 2012, from www.holbrookstreetpress.com/ptsd-can-attack-years-later.php

Kellett, R. (2012). Classes and games help kids experiencing post-earthquake trauma. Retrieved August 10, 2012, from www.mercycorps.org/countries/iran/10325

Kerig, P., & Becker, S. (2010). From internalizing to externalizing: Theoretical models of the processes linking PTSD to juvenile delinquency. In S. J. Egan (Ed.), *Post-Traumatic stress disorder: Causes, symptoms, and treatment*. Hauppage, NY: Nova Science.

Klein, R., & Klein, N. (2011). *Relaxation and success imagery* (CD). Retrieved from http://www.innercoaching.com

Kross, E., Berman, M., Mischel, W., Smith, E., & Wager, T. (2011). Social rejection shares somatosensory representations with physical pain. *Proceedings of the National Academy of Sciences*, published online before print March 28, 2011. doi: 10.1073/pnas.1102693108 http://www.pnas.org/content/early/2011/03/22/1102693108.full.pdf+html

Kuban, C. (2008). *One-minute interventions: For traumatized children and adolescents*. Clinton Township, MI: TLC Institute.

Kuban, C. (2009). *A time for resilience*. Clinton Township, MI: TLC Institute.

Lakes, K. D., & Hoyt, W. T. (2004). Promoting self-regulation through school-based martial arts training. *Applied Developmental Psychology, 25*, 283–302.

Langmuir, J., Kirsch, S., & Classen, C. (2012). A pilot study of body-oriented group psychotherapy: Adapting sensorimotor psychotherapy for the group treatment of trauma, *Psychological Trauma: Theory, Research Practice, and Policy, 4*(2), 214–220.

Laursen, E. (2008). Respectful alliances. *Reclaiming Children and Youth, 17*(1), 4–9.

LeDoux, J. (2002). *Synoptic self: How our brains become who we are*. New York, NY: Penguin.

Levine, P. A., & Kline, M. (2007). *Trauma through a child's eyes: Awakening the ordinary miracle of healing*. Berkeley, CA: North Atlantic Books.

Levine, P. A., & Kline, M. (2008). *Trauma-proofing your kids: A parents' guide for instilling confidence, joy, and resilience*. Berkeley, CA: North Atlantic Books.

Levine, S. Z., Laufer, A., Hamama-Raz, Y., Stein, E., & Solomon, Z. (2008). Posttraumatic growth in adolescence: Examining its components and relationship with PTSD. *Journal of Traumatic Stress, 21*(5), 492–496.

Lieberman, A., Van Horn, P., & Ozer, E. (2005). The impact of domestic violence on preschoolers: Predictive and mediating factors. *Developmental Psychopathology, 17*(2), 385–396.

Linehan, M. M., Bohus, M., & Lynch, M. (2010). Dialetical behavior therapy for pervasive dysregulation. In J. Groos (Ed.), *Handbook of emotional regulation* (pp. 581–605). New York, NY: Guilford Press.

Lonigan, C., Shannon, M., Finch, A., Daugherty, T., & Taylor, C. (1991). Children's reactions to a natural disaster: Symptom severity and degree of exposure. *Advances in Behavior Research and Therapy, 13*, 135–154.

Looks like another Black Monday. (2008, September 30). *Wall Street Journal*, p. C6.

Magwaza, A., Killian, B., Peterson, I., & Pillay, Y. (1993). The effects of chronic stress on preschool children living in South African townships. *Child Abuse and Neglect, 17*, 795–803.

Malchiodi, C. A. (1990). *Breaking the silence*. New York, NY: Brunner/Mazel.

Malchiodi, C. A. (2008). Creative interventions and childhood trauma. In C. Malchiodi (Ed.), *Creative interventions with traumatized children* (pp. 3–21). New York, NY: Guilford Press.

Martin, L. (2002). *Invisible table: Reflections on youth and youth work in New Zealand*. Albany, NY: Thomson Learning.

Maslow, A. (1954). *Motivation and personality*. New York NY: Harper & Row.

McFarlane, A., Policansky, S., & Irwin, C. (1987). A longitudinal study of the psychological morbidity in children due to a natural disaster. *Psychological Medicine, 17*, 727–738.

Michaesu, G., & Baettig, D. (1996). An integrated model of post-traumatic stress disorder. *The European Journal of Psychiatry, 10*(4), 233–242.

Mitchell, M., Brendtro, L., Jackson, C., & Foltz. R. (2012). *Comparison between deficit thinking and strength-based thinking*. Albion, MI: Starr Commonwealth.

Morris, B. A., Shakespeare-Finch, J. E., & Scott, J. L. (2007). Coping processes and dimensions of posttraumatic growth. *The Australasian Journal of Disaster and Trauma Studies, 1*, 1–12.

Nader, K. (2008). *Understanding and assessing trauma in children and adolescents*. New York, NY: Routledge.

National Center for Trauma-Informed Care (NCTIC). (2011). *What's trauma-informed care?* Retrieved June 30, 2011, from www.samhsa.gov/nctic/trauma.asp

National Child Traumatic Stress Network (NCTSN). (2005). *Mental health interventions for refugee children in resettlement* (White Paper II). Los Angeles, CA: National Child Traumatic Stress Network.

National Victims of Crime. (2004) *Assessing resilience*. Retrieved May 22, 2012, from www.ncvc .org/ncvc/main.aspx?dblD=DB_Bibliograph110

Newman, T. (2004). *What works for building resilience*. Retrieved May 3, 2012, from www .barnardos.org.uk/what_works_in_building_resilience_summary_1_.pdf

Oehlberg, B. (2006). *Reaching and teaching stressed and anxious learners*. Thousand Oaks, CA: Corwin Press.

Ogden, P., Minton, K., & Pain, C. (2006). *Trauma and the body: A sensorimotor approach to psychotherapy*. New York, NY: W. W. Norton.

Olafson, E., & Kenniston, J. (2008). Obtaining information from children in the justice system. *Juvenile and Family Court Journal, 59*(4), 71–89.

Osofsky, J. (Ed.). (2004). *Young children and trauma*. New York, NY: Guilford Press.

Ovaert, L. B., Cashel, M. L., & Sewell, K. W. (2003). Structured group therapy for posttraumatic stress disorder in incarcerated male juveniles. *American Journal of Orthopsychiatry, 2*, 294–301.

Padesky, C. A. (1993). *Socratic questioning: Changing minds or guiding discovery?* A keynote address delivered on September 24, 1993, at the European Congress of Behavioral and Cognitive Therapies, London, England.

Perry, B. D. (2004). *Children & loss*. Retrieved October 20, 2004, from http://teacher.scholastic .com/professional/bruceperry/childrenloss.htm

Perry, B. D. (2005). *Bruce Perry on play*. Retrieved December 7, 2012, from http://infanttoddler specialistgroup.com/?p=293

Perry, B. (2012) Creating an emotionally safe classroom. Retrieved August 10, 2012, from http://teacher.scholastic.com/professional/bruceperry/safety_wonder.htm

Perry, B. D. (2009). Examining child maltreatment through a neurodevelopmental lens: Clinical applications of the neurosequential model of therapeutics. *Journal of Loss and Trauma, 14*(4), 16.

Perry, B. D., & Hambrick, E. (2008). The neurosequential model of therapeutics. *Reclaiming Children and Youth, 17*(3), 38–43.

Perry, B. D., & Szalavitz, M. (2006). *The boy who was raised as a dog, and other stories from a child psychiatrist's notebook.* New York, NY: Basic Books.

Philipsen, G. (1992). Recent books in qualitative research methodology. *Communication Education, 41*, 240–245.

Punamäki, R.-L., Qouta, S., Miller, T., & El-Sarra, E. (2011). Who are the resilient children in the presence of military violence? *Journal of Peace Psychology, 17*(4), 389–416.

Pynoos, R., & Eth, S. (1986). Witness to violence: The child interview. *Journal of the American Academy of Child Psychiatry, 25*, 306–319.

Pynoos, R., Frederick, C., Nader, K., Arroyo, E., Steinberg, A., Eth, S., Nunez, F., & Fairbanks, L. (1987). Life threat and posttraumatic stress in school-age children. *Archives in General Psychiatry, 44*, 1057–1063.

Pynoos, R. S., Aisenberg, E., Layne, C. M., Saltzman, W. R., & Steinberg, A. M. (2001). School-based trauma and grief intervention for adolescents. *The Prevention Researcher, 10*, 3.

Raider, M., & Steele, W. (2010). Structured sensory therapy (SITCAP-ART) for traumatized adjudicated adolescents in residential treatment. *National Social Sciences Journal, 32*(1), 111–121.

Raider, M., Steele, W., & Kuban, C. (2012). A school-based trauma program for elementary school children. *Naitonal Social Sciences Journal, 39*, 65–86.

Ramachandran, V. (2011). *The tell-tale brain: A neuroscientist's quest for what makes us human.* New York, NY: W. W. Norton.

Rankin, J. R., & Gilligan, T. D. (2004). Resiliency: How can you help your students bounce back from life's bumps? *Virginia's Journal of Education, 98*(1), 11–15.

Riley, S. (1997). Children's art and narratives: An opportunity to enhance therapy and a supervisory challenge. *The Supervision Bulletin, 9*, 2–3.

Riley, S. (2001). *Group process made visible: Group art therapy.* New York, NY: Routledge.

Roje, J. (1995). LA '94 earthquake in the eyes of the children: Art therapy with elementary school children who were victims of the disaster. *Art Therapy: Journal of the American Art therapy Association, 12*, 237–243.

Roma, L., & Segura, D. (2010). Enhancing the resilience of young single mothers of colour: A review of programs and services. *Journal of Education for Students Placed at Risk, 15*, 173–185.

Rothschild, B. (2000). *The body remembers: The psychophysiology of trauma and trauma treatment.* New York, NY: W. W. Norton.

Rothschild, B. (2011). An open letter to visitors of Babette's website. Retrieved on March 20, 2011, from http://home.webuniverse.net/babette/

Saigh, P., & Bremner, J. (1999). *Posttraumatic stress disorder.* Boston, MA: Allyn and Bacon.

Scaer, R. (2005). *The trauma spectrum: Hidden wounds and hidden resiliency.* New York, NY: W. W. Norton.

Scales, P., & Leffert, N. (2004). *Developmental assets: A synthesis of the scientific research on adolescent development* (2nd ed.). Minneapolis, MN: The Search Institute.

Schedl, M. (2010). Nightmares: An underdiagnosed and untreated condition? *Sleep, 33*(6), 733–734.

Schore, A. (2001). The effects of a secure attachment relationship on right-brain development, affect regulation, and infant mental health. *Infant Mental Health Journal, 22*(1–2), 7–66.

Science 20 (News Staff). (2009, March 12). *Art therapy? Drawing enhances emotional verbalization, say researchers.* Retrieved March 3, 2012, from www.science20.com/news_releases/ art_therapy_drawing_enhances_emotional_verbalization_say_researchers

Seligman, M. (1990*). Learned optimism: How to change your mind and your life.* New York, NY: Free Press.

Shelden, D., Angell, M., Stoner, J., & Roseland, B. (2010). School principal's influence on trust: Perspectives of mothers of children with disabilities. *The Journal of Educational Research, 103* (3), 159–170.

Sheppard, L. (1998). *Brave Bart: A story for traumatized and grieving children.* Clinton Township, MI: TLC Institute.

Shirk, S., & Karver, M. S. (2003). Prediction of treatment outcome from relationship variables in child and adolescent therapy: A meta-analytic review. *Journal of Consulting and Clinical Psychology, 71*(3), 452–464.

Siegel, D. (1999). *The developing mind.* New York, NY: Guilford Press.

Siegel, D. (2003). An interpersonal neurobiology of psychotherapy: The developing mind and the resolution of trauma. In M. Solomon & D. Siegel (Eds.), *Healing trauma: Attachment, mind, body, and brain* (pp. 1–5). New York, NY: W. W. Norton.

Siegel, D. (2007). *The mindful brain: Reflections and attunement in the cultivation of well-being.* New York, NY: W. W. Norton.

Smith, J. (2012). *Integrative psychotherapy.* Retrieved March 6, 2012, from www.psytx.com/ 03sessions.html

Snowden, L. R., Hu, T., & Jerrell, M. (1995). Emergency care avoidance: Ethnic matching and participation in minority-serving program. *Community Mental Health Journal, 31*(5), 463–473.

Sohn, A., & Grayson, C. (2005). *Parenting your Asperger child: Individualized solutions for teaching your child practical skills.* New York, NY: Perigee Trade.

Solomon, Z., & Dekel, R. (2007). Posttraumatic stress disorder and posttraumatic growth among Israeli ex-POWs. *Journal of Traumatic Stress, 20*(3), 303–312.

Spreet, D. (2009). *Fear and posttramatic stress disorder.* Retrieved February 14, 2012, from www .brainfacts.org/across-the-lifespan/stress-and-anxiety/articles/2009

Starkman, P. A., Gebarski, M. N., Berent, S. S., & Schteingart, D. E. (1992). Hippocampal formation volume, memory of dysfunction and cortisol levels in patients with Cushing's syndrome. *Biology Psychiatry, 32*, 756–765.

Steele, W. (2003). Using drawing in short-term trauma resolution. In C. Malchiodi (Ed.), *Handbook of art therapy* (pp. 139–151). New York, NY: Guilford Press.

Steele, W., & Kuban, C. (2011). Trauma-informed resilience and post-traumatic growth (PTG). *Reclaiming Children and Youth, 20*(3), 44–46.

Steele, W., Kuban, C., & Raider, L. M. (2009). Connections, continuity, dignity, opportunities model: Follow-up of children who completed the I Feel Better Now! trauma intervention program. *School Social Work Journal, 33*(2), 98–111.

Steele, W., & Malchiodi, M. (2012). *Trauma-informed practices with children and adolescents.* New York, NY: Routledge Taylor & Francis.

Steele, W., Malchiodi, M., & Kline, N. (2002). *Helping children feel safe.* Clinton Township, MI: TLC Institute.

Steele, W., & Raider, M. (2001). *Structured sensory interventions for children, adolescents and parents (SITCAP).* New York, NY: Edwin Mellen Press.

Steele, W., Raider, M., Delillo-Storey, M., Jacobs, J., & Kuban, C. (2008). Structured sensory therapy (SITCAP-ART) for traumatized adjudicated adolescents in residential treatment. *Residential Treatment for Children and Youth, 25*(2), 167–185.

Stien, P. T., & Kendall, J. C. (2004). *Psychological trauma and the developing brain: Neurologically based interventions for troubled children.* New York, NY: Routledge.

Straussner, S. L., & Phillips, N. K. (2004). *Understanding mass violence: A social work perspective.* Boston, MA: Allyn & Bacon.

Stubner, M., Nader, K., Yasuda, P., Pynoos, R., & Cohen, S. (1991). Stress responses after pediatric bone-marrow transplantation: Preliminary results of a prospective longitudinal study. *Journal of the American Academy of Child and Adolescent Psychiatry, 30,* 952–957.

Stuttered Speech Syndrome: Advancing the understanding of stuttering. (2012). Retrieved May 1, 2012, from www.stutteredspeechsyndrome.com

Sweatt, J. D. (2009). *Mechanisms of memory.* Waltham, MA: Academic Press.

Tate, T., & Copas, R. (2010). "Peer pressure" and the group process: Building cultures of concern. *Reclaiming Children and Youth, 19*(1), 12–16.

Taylor, M. (1999). *Imaginary companions and the children who create them.* New York, NY: Oxford University Press.

Tedeschi, R. G., & Calhoun, L. (2004). Posttraumatic growth: Conceptual foundations and empirical evidence. *Psychological Inquiry, 15*(1), 1–18.

Tedeschi, R. G., & Kilmer, R. P. (2005). Assessing strengths, resilience, and growth to guide clinical interventions. *Professional Psychology: Research and Practice, 36*(3), 230–237.

Tedeschi, R. G., Park, C. L., & Calhoun, L. G. (1998). Posttraumatic growth: Conceptual issues. In R. G. Tedeschi, C. L. Park, & L. G. Calhoun (Eds.), *Posttraumatic growth: Positive changes in the aftermath of crisis* (pp. 1–22). Mahwah, NJ: Erlbaum.

Teicher, M. (2000). Wounds that time won't heal: The neurobiology of child abuse. *Cerebrum: The Dana Forum on Brain Sciences, 2,* 50–68.

Terr, L. (1990). *Too scared to cry.* New York, NY: Harper & Row.

Terr, L. (1994). *Unchained memories.* New York, NY: Basic Books.

Terr, L. (2008). *Magical moments of change: How psychotherapy turns kids around.* New York, NY: W. W. Norton.

Terr, L. C. (1979). Children of Chowchilla study of psychic trauma. *Psychoanalytic Study of the Child, 34,* 547–623.

Thomas, E. (2009). Author entry. Retrieved May 15, 2012, from http://en.wikipedia.org/wiki/Ed_Thomas

Turner, D., & Cox, H. (2004). Facilitating posttraumatic growth. *Health and Quality of Life Outcome, 2,* 43.

Unger, M., Brown, M., Liedenburg, L., Cheung, M., & Levine, K. (2008). Distinguishing differences in pathways to resilience among Canadian youth. *Canadian Journal Community Mental Health, 27,* 1–3.

Van Bockern, S., & McDonald, T. (2012). Creating Circle of Courage schools. *Reclaiming Children and Youth, 20*(4), 13–17.

Van Dalen, A. (2001). Juvenile violence and addiction: Tangle roots in childhood trauma. *Journal of Social Work Practice in the Addictions, 1,* 25–40.

van der Kolk, B. A. (1994). The body keeps the score: Memory and the evolving psychobiology of posttraumatic stress. *Harvard Review of Psychiatry, 1*(5), 253–265.

van der Kolk, B. A. (2005). Developmental trauma. *Psychiatric Annals, 35,* 401.

van der Kolk, B. A. (2006). Clinical implications of neuroscience research in PTSD. *Annals of the New York Academy of Sciences, 1,* 1–17.

van der Kolk, B. A., McFarlane, A. C., & Weisaeth, L. (Eds.). (1996). *Traumatic stress: The effects of overwhelming experience on mind, body, and society.* New York, NY: Guilford Press.

van der Kolk, B. A., Pynoos, R. S., Cicchetti, D., Cloitre, M., D'Andrea, W., Ford, J. D., . . . Teicher, M. (2009). Proposal to include a developmental trauma disorder diagnosis for children and adolescents in DSM-V. Official submission from the National Child Traumatic Stress Network Developmental Trauma Disorder Taskforce to the American Psychiatric Association.

Walsh, D. (2012). *School-based supports for students with depression.* Retrieved January 2, 2012, from http://udini.proquest.com/view/school-based-supports-for-pqid:2329754231/

Webb, N. (1986). Before and after suicide: A preventive outreach program for colleges. *Suicide and Life-Threatening Behavior, 16*(4), 469–480.

Weinberger, D. A. (1990). The construct validity of the repressive coping style. In J. L. Singer (Ed.), *Repression and dissociation: Implications for personality theory, psychopathology, and health* (pp. 337–386). Chicago, IL: University of Chicago Press.

Weinberger, D. A., Schwartz, G. E., & Davidson, R. J. (1979). Low-anxious, high-anxious, and repressive coping styles: Psychometric patterns and behavioral and physiological responses to stress. *Journal of Abnormal Psychology, 88,* 369–380.

Weinhold, J. B., & Weinhold, B. K. (2009). *Developmental trauma.* Retrieved October 23, 2012, from www.weinholds.org/main/

Werner, E. E. (2012). Risk, resilience, and recovery. *Reclaiming Children and Youth, 21*(1).

Werner, E. E., & Smith, R. S. (1992). *Overcoming the odds: High-risk children from birth to adulthood.* Ithaca, NY: Cornell University Press.

Werner, E. E., & Smith, R. S. (2001). *Journey from childhood to midlife: Resilience and recovery.* Ithaca, NY: Cornell University Press.

Werner, S. R. (1989). *Vulnerable but invincible: A longitudinal study of resilient children and youth.* New York, NY: Adams, Banister, Cox. (Original work published 1982.)

Witness Justice. (2010). *Trauma is the common denominator: New discoveries in the science of traumatic behavior.* Retrieved from www.witnessjustice.org/resources/trauma.cfm

Wolin, S., & Wolin, S. J. (2000). Shifting paradigms: Easier said than done. *Strength Based Services Intervention Newsletter,* 1–4.

World Health Organization (WHO). (2012). *International classification of diseases (ICD-10)* (10th ed.). Retrieved January 6, 2012, from www.who.int/classification/icd/en/

Yellin, P. B. (2012). 3 Keys to Foster Resilience in Children with LD and ADHD. Retrieved November 31, 2012, from www.smartkidswithld.org/ld-basics/beyond-the-classroom/3-keys-to-foster-resilience-withld-adhd.html

Yule, W. (1992). Post-traumatic stress disorder in child survivors of shipping disasters: The sinking of the Jupiter. *Psychotherapy and Psychosomatics, 57*(4), 200–205.

Ziegler, D. (2002). *Traumatic experience and the brain: A handbook for understanding and treating those traumatized as children.* Phoenix, AZ: Acacia.

Author Index

Subject Index